To Teach a Dyslexic

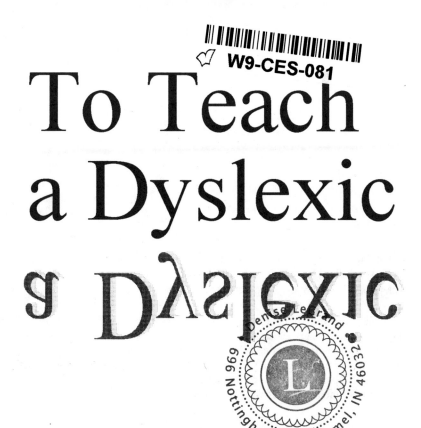

A Dyslexic Tells How Luck Enabled
Him to Learn to Read...
& How His Blissful Ignorance &
Stubbornness Enabled Him To
Discover How to Teach Other
Dyslexics to Read and Write

Don McCabe

2

Library of Congress Cataloging in Publication Data

McCabe, Don
  To teach a dyslexic.
  Includes index and glossary.
  1. Dyslexia. 2. Learning disabilities. 3. Learning disabled children. 4.
McCabe, Don. 5. Teachers of handicapped children –United States – Biography.
6. Teachers of dyslexic children – United States – Biography.
I. Title.
Library of Congress Classification Number: LC4704.L96
Library of Congress Card Numer: To be determined
Dewey Decimal Classification Number:
ISBN: 1-56400-004-4

Printed in the United States of America

P .١٢٨

To the fond memory of my sister Betty June Szilagyi
who was my first and by far my most
important teacher

Once there was a fiddler who played with so much rhythm and excitement that everybody just had to dance.

One day a deaf mute stopped by. He had never heard of music. He had never heard of dancing.

What he saw was a man on a stage pumping one foot up and down, holding a funny wooden box under his chin, and running a stick across it.

He also saw the people around him were throwing their arms up and down and wiggling their butts and in general behaving like lunatics in an asylum.

To the deaf mute, what he saw was senseless and in bad taste.

> —An Hasidic parable with apologies to Martin Buber whose translation of that parable was such exquisite poetry that I can honestly say, it was the only poetry that was immediately and indelibly etched upon my memory.
> I admit to changing it to what my editors consider a more readily understandable prose. If you ever can find his book *Tales of the Hasidim,* read it in its original.

Which part of this book should you read first?

- If your interest lies mainly in finding out what dyslexia really is and how best to "identify," treat, or "prevent" dyslexia start with chapter 16.

- If you are interested in finding out **_why_** it took a dyslexic to do what thousands of more learned individuals in universities could not or would not do, start from the very beginning and enjoy!

- If you are primarily concerned with **_helping_** a specific individual such as your son, daughter, husband, or wife, skip to chapter 19.

But at least read the chapter titles
to see what you will be missing.
You can always come back
later and read them.

Contents

Part I – The why of my dyslexia, and how it was overcome:

Part II – Twists and turns of fate that prepared and led a dyslexic into teaching dyslexics and finding out what dyslexia is all about:

Part III — Educational Research: In what direction/s should AVKO go?

Part IV – Suggestions to public or private school systems and home-schoolers

Part V – Chapters I haven't written, but might get around to writing someday.

27. Beware of educational studies. You can find studies to support almost any viewpoint. Learn how to do your own. . . . . . .

28. Beware of major school book publishers. There may not be a conspiracy as such, but the very nature of publishing and marketing encourages a situation that is educationally unhealthy. . . . .

29. How the federal and state departments of education waste tons of money. . . . .

30. A Practical Use for Miscue Analysis: Building self-esteem*[1]

31. Learning about the learning-to-read and learning-to-write process by teaching yourself how to read upside down and to write upside down and mirror image with your other hand.*

32. Comprehension and Schema theory: a practical use* . . . . .

33. Underlining—Cuing the computer brain* . . . .

34. The SQ3R reading formula really works* . . . .

35. 220 names/faces; 220 Dolch sight words are 200 too many for students with memories like mine* . . . .

---

[1]Items marked with the little star or asterisk (*) are available now in pamphlet form from the AVKO Foundation.

The Appendix – Miscellaneous items that might be of interest to some people, but certainly not to all.

Author's Foreword

Damn it Don, get dressed.

"DAMN IT, DON! Get dressed! I'm taking you into the hospital right now." My wife Ann never swears. Well, almost never. So when she spoke to me like that at 3 AM January 12th, 1992 I just said, "Yes, dear" and got dressed. I felt *something* was wrong with me, but I knew it just *couldn't* be my heart. After all, I knew all the symptoms. I wasn't having any chest pains. I had no numbness. I wasn't sick to my stomach. I just couldn't get comfortable. I just couldn't get to sleep. If I didn't have the symptoms, I couldn't be having a heart attack. That was simple logic—the same simple straight forward logic that dyslexics use when trying to read or spell. That logic, accepting as 100% true what is given by experts (in the case of dyslexia, teachers) or in my case, doctors, and then applying that logic almost killed me.

Thank God, Ann is not a dyslexic. She learned early to disregard statements by teachers about sounds and spellings when they didn't work. She never has cared that the *sound* "fish" is rarely spelled *fish*. She just automatically, unconsciously, substitutes *fici* for the spelling of the sound "fish" when she spells *official* or *beneficial* but uses *fish* in *fisheries*. Just as she has trusted her instincts rather than logic in learning to read and spell, she trusted her instincts and thumbed her nose at my logic. She just knew I was having a heart attack.

So when we got there, Ann told me to tell the attendants I was having chest pains. I wasn't. But who am I to argue with my wife. So I said I was having chest pains. And almost like on TV in rushed doctors and nurses and I was quickly hooked up to a monitor. They started hanging IV's and asked me if I were allergic to any medications and was I on any medication. Easy questions for me to answer with, "No." Then I heard the physician on duty say to the young interns as he pointed to the monitor, "Now that's what a major heart attack looks like!" Then the legal spiel ensued about using clot busters. I just said if I'm having a heart attack, go ahead and use them. They did.

They managed to stop the attack and to get my heart functioning almost normally. Normal was out of the question because there was some serious blockage. I had my choice of angioplasty (the balloon), by-pass, or the new laser plus angioplasty. After having consulted several physicians and cardiologists, I went with the latter and had Dr. Daniel Anbe, the head of cardiology at McLaren Hospital in Flint perform the honors.

Now I wasn't his first patient to have this type of surgery, but I was his first (and probably last) to have the surgery while wearing a beret. Because I'm bald and because in the hospital's own literature about what to do after a heart attack they said you should keep your head covered, I held them to their word. If they don't provide head coverings the same way they do foot coverings, I ought to be able to provide my own. A dyslexic's logic is impeccable and usually works.

It was the heart attack that made me realize that I couldn't be sure as to how much time I would have left to finish my work. So I have been doing three things. One, I have slowed down my pace. Two, I've been watching my diet. And three, I have been finishing my work and writing an autobiography in hopes that the academic world will somehow be forced into looking at what I have done and finally come to understand, that just as it might take a thief to catch a thief, it also might take a dyslexic to teach teachers how to teach dyslexics.

Thank God for ignorance
and a loving family

THAT I CAN READ and write is really a small miracle. If I had been born in 1972 instead of 1932, there's no doubt in my mind I would be illiterate today.

But sometimes, ignorance can be bliss. The doctor who delivered me kept my parents ignorant of my condition. According to my mother, who happened to be present at my birth, I didn't want to come into this world. At least not head first.

It was about 3 P.M. on October 4, 1932, exactly twenty-five years before Sputnik that I arrived into this world, blue and bloody with the umbilical cord wrapped around my neck. I had presented my posterior first which the doctor did not appreciate. He had no sense of humor. He didn't like being mooned. But he managed to turn me around with forceps and extract me while doing a real number on my mother's birth canal.

It being in the depths of the BIG DEPRESSION, there weren't many nurses on duty. Would you believe my father was called into the delivery room? Today, it might be almost routine for a father to witness a birth. Then, it wasn't. In fact, my dad never saw my birth. He was just called in because the doctor needed all the help he could get from nurses to save my mother's life. She was hemorrhaging badly.

According to my dad, the doctor handed me to him with a very simple instruction: "Clean the gunk out of his mouth and see if you can get him breathing." Well, my dad followed the instructions. He got me breathing.

Afterwards, the doctor never bothered to tell my parents that because of the extremely difficult delivery and being born blue, that I had suffered oxygen deprivation and was probably brain damaged. They do that now, routinely. Then, they didn't. Thank God.

But it was more than my parents' ignorance of my condition that enabled me to learn to read, to excel in school, and to eventually become a member of *Who's Who in Education*. I was their third child with four more yet to come. So they already had some experience in child rearing.

Without realizing it they practiced what is now generally called "intensive stimulation." This method of treating Down's syndrome children (or Mongolian idiots as they were called when I was growing up) frequently allows these children to develop into reasonably normal literate adults.

Thank God for ignorance and great expectations. My parents loved children. They loved to see them laugh. They loved to see them eat and grow. They loved to talk to them, sing to them, dance with them, play with them. They just *knew* when children were supposed to be able to walk and talk. About nine months. My older brother Jack did. My older sister Betty June did. And all my younger brothers and sisters, Tom, Mary, Nan, and Jim did. Me? Well, I was the slowest of the seven. I was brain damaged. Remember? Well, I was two days away from being 10 months old when I took my first steps.

Why was I, a brain-damaged child, able to walk this early? Simple. I was constantly receiving physical therapy. That's not what my parents, my older brother and sister, and my grandparents would have called it. They simply would have called it play. They played with me. From the start they would extend a finger for each of my hands to grab. They would tug. I would tug back reflexively. That's exercise. That's physical therapy. But to my shanty Irish family, it was just playing with the baby.

My grandmother told me that I was the crankiest baby in the whole McCabe-Webb tribe. But they never let me just lie there and cry. They didn't just stick me in a crib and tuck me away in a room and close a door. No. Someone would always pick me up and change my diaper, feed me, burp me, sing to and dance with me. Music. Rhythm. Love. Words being sung. Tone of voice showing love. Giving attention. Giving physical exercise. Praise for the smallest of physical achievements whether it was lifting my head or reaching out or grabbing a finger. It's true I can't remember that. But I do remember how my two younger brothers and two younger sisters were treated. And when I was a sophomore in college and had to write an autobiography for my child psychology class, I did a rather extensive interview with my parents. And I interviewed my Grandma and Grandpa Webb. Separately. For they were separated.

I never did understand that as a child. Either Grandma or Grandpa was always around. But excepting for Christmas they were never together in our house. And when they were, they never shared the same bedroom. They were loving grandparents. And never did I ever hear either of them say anything bad about the other. We kids always hoped they would get back together. I know I prayed for that. And so did my older sister Betty June. How could we know then that Grandma was a quite a feminist for her day? How could we know then that grandpa was what we call today a male chauvinist who considered wife-beating as a man's natural God-given prerogative sanctioned by the church and state. Grandma disagreed. I was almost thirty years old before I learned the truth about Grandma and Grandpa Webb.

In a way I'm lucky that we were poor. There was hardly enough money for food and clothes. There wasn't any for baby toys. No fancy plastic rattles for me or mobiles to watch spinning endlessly around. No baby buggy. No training wheels called a walker that delay and interfere with learning balance. But I had clothespins and small tin pots to make into drums to beat on with my spoons. I had no crib. When I was too big for a dresser drawer, I slept with my parents and then in a small hand-built bunk bed in a room with my older brother and sister. I was never really left alone.

I had no playpen. Thank God. Today when I see a child sitting in a playpen I'm reminded of monkeys in cages in a zoo. I crawled. I climbed. I toddled. I got into cupboards. I got into trouble. But I was loved. I was played with. Especially by my older sister Betty June.

Betty always wanted to play school. She always wanted to play teacher. Guess who her student was? So whatever she was learning in kindergarten she tried to teach me. I'm just two years old, but she's teaching me to play with crayons. To color mostly on paper but often on walls. To write. Now, she wasn't the best kindergarten student. In fact, she flunked kindergarten. She claimed she just was held back. But I always prefer saying she flunked. It makes for better story telling when I tell my audiences that she ended up making the 1951 *Who's Who in American Colleges and Universities.*

From Betty I learned early to use my fingers. I drew. I colored. I cut out paper dolls. All before I went to school. My older brother Jack didn't have many kids his age to play with. So when he wanted to play catch, he had me. He was a patient teacher, too. And good. But then again, our dad was quite an athlete in his day. And Jack not only inherited some of his athletic ability but was taught by him. How good was he? Well, in a minor league exhibition game, our dad pitched a three-hitter against Satchel Paige. He lost 1-0. But then again, who didn't lose against Satchel?

If I had to pick the one best teacher I ever had, it would be a hard choice between my older sister Betty June and my Grandpa Webb. But Betty June would be my pick. She played school with me and tried to teach me what she was learning in school. She taught me to play jacks, hopscotch, paper dolls, and just plain dolls. Grandpa Webb taught me to gamble.

Well, not at first. You see Grandpa Webb was quite a character to say the least. He was part American Indian (most likely Chippewa), part French, and part Irish as near as I can tell. One thing he was really good at was cards. Today, he might be considered a professional gambler. Then, he just liked to play cards now and then to supplement his income. But in the afternoons there wasn't a lot of action. So he would play solitaire.

Little two or three-year-old Donnie liked to watch. An observer might have used the word *pester* to describe what I did. At any rate, Grandpa Webb would give me a battered old deck to play with when he played. To keep me occupied, he first taught me to build houses out of cards. Then eventually, he taught me how to play solitaire when I was about four. By the time I was five he had taught me how to play knock rummy.

What a natural teacher he was. My older brother Jack didn't like the way Grandpa taught me. Grandpa always sat to my right. And if I played correctly, he saw to it that I won. Jack never did like losing to me. Still doesn't as a matter of fact. But Grandpa tried to make sure Jack won some too, but if he won two cents, I would always win three. Thanks to Grandpa.

How was I to know that he could look into my hand anytime he wanted to? I was just a little five-year-old.

And we played for pennies. Well, not really. My mother had pretensions of being lace curtain Irish. She would not tolerate teaching children to gamble with money. So Grandpa used match sticks. Of course, shades of Piaget and his principle of conservation, these were converted to pennies after we finished the game and when my mother wasn't watching.

Grandpa was a natural teacher. If I picked up to make a pair, I lost. And he wouldn't let me search through the discard pile. "If you want to hunt, take a hound and go north" was his favorite saying. Somehow or another no matter how long we played, I always won at least a penny. Sometimes as many as four. Great confidence builder Grandpa was. But he wasn't afraid to let me get behind. Once I owed him six cents. I had to play hard to get back to even because I didn't have any money to pay him if we quit right then.

Today in special education the experts talk about the need for manipulatives to teach math. Well, my grandpa was great with manipulatives. Cards. Matches. Pennies. Nickels. Dimes, even. He didn't know it, but he built for me a solid foundation in mathematics long before I had them in school. It was done slowly. It was done having fun. What a great teacher. Lousy husband to my Grandma Webb and certainly not a great father to his own kids, but a great, great grandpa to me.

My other grandparents I rarely saw. They lived too far away. By the time gasoline rationing and World War II ended, they both were dead, so I have only vague memories of them. But for some reason I had a strong memory of their dog "Mustard." Not until recently, when I was reminiscing with my cousin Georgia who knew them well, did I realize they didn't have a dog "Mustard." The dog's name was Buster. Dyslexic hearing. As a child I hadn't known any Buster's, but I knew what mustard was. Apparently the sounds of "Buster" that entered my ears were changed into something more recognizable by my dyslexic computer brain. Later on, I discovered that this dyslexic phenomenon is shared by almost everybody. In chapter 24 I tell how I stumbled onto a way to prove our computer brains, whether dyslexic or not, are programmed to change what our senses detect to fit our inner concept of reality.

Chapter 2

Thank God for Cook School

and great expectations

BUT EVEN WITH THE great head start I had at home, I still probably would never have learned to read and write if it hadn't have been for the fact that our house was on a block that had been gerrymandered into the Cook School district.

Flint, Michigan at that time was under the complete dominance of General Motors. GM ran the town. GM ran the school board. GM looked out for the best interests of its executives. GM had bought a number of houses in the Cook School area so that when it transferred executives into the city they would have a place to live within walking distance of a good grade school. And Cook School wasn't just good. It was great.

Mrs. McLeod was the principal. Mrs. Brown taught kindergarten. Mrs. Carpenter taught first grade. All the teachers were good. They had to be good teachers to be assigned to Cook School. Just how good a school was Cook with its thirty to thirty five students per grade? When I graduated in 1950, *The Flint Journal* printed the names and pictures not only of the valedictorians and salutatorians but of all those who graduated magna and summa cum laude in the three public high schools in Flint as well as the four smaller parochial high schools. All my classmates were there. Well, almost all. Little Annabelle Dillon, my kindergarten sweetheart, didn't make it. The rest did. In fact, the valedictorian from Flint Central was Willie Parkinson. The valedictorian from Flint Northern was Robert Richardson. Or was it Richard Robertson. I forget. I do remember I was the salutatorian from Flint Technical. What are the odds, you mathematicians, for one little grade school out of about twenty grade schools monopolizing all the honors?

Had I lived across the street I would have gone to Doyle where most of the transients went to school. One block north and I would have had to go to Dort. Dort wasn't a bad school, but it was far from being the great grade school that Cook was.

I lived one block east of Detroit Street. Today this street is called Martin Luther King, Jr. Blvd. But back then it was Detroit Street. It was a natural dividing line. West of Detroit Street was where the professionals lived. That was where many G.M. executives lived. So I went to school with rich kids. At least they seemed rich to me. They all had money to buy candy at Eli's Grocery Store across from Cook School. I didn't. They all had real nice homes, toys and games to play with. I didn't. They got a dollar for every A on their report card. I didn't get a penny. But I did have Grandpa and Grandma. And I had two great parents that made up for their lack of money with lots of love and attention. I had Betty June who played teacher. I had Jack who was my coach. He taught me to run. I had to. He chased me many a time and generally for good reason. I wasn't the nicest little brother. I had a bad temper and a penchant for throwing things at him from stones to a piano bench one time. He didn't take kindly to that. And I hated to get caught by him.

But Jack still needed me if only for him to practice throwing a football or baseball. And I was a tag-along. When he went to play ball in the vacant lot, there I was. I played with my brother's friends who were three to six years older than I was. Good practice. That type of physical development enabled me to always be a little better than my classmates. They were rich kids. I was shanty Irish from the wrong side of Detroit St. From day one, I was the toughest kid in my class. And the teachers expected that of me. They also expected that I would be the smartest.

Talk about expectations. My brother Jack was an all-A student at Cook. He was captain of the Patrol Boys, captain of the softball and soccer team, and winner of the 50-yard-dash. Betty June was an all-A student and she won the girls' 50-yard-dash. And she never let Jack or me forget that her time was one tenth of a second better than ours.

I had the same teachers that Jack and Betty had. The teachers knew I was a little different than Jack and Betty. I couldn't sit still. I always had to be doing something. But instead of punishing me, they made use of my energy. I was put in charge of all kinds of things. Especially in kindergarten.

My first grade teacher, Mrs. Carpenter, had no training in handling students with Attention Deficit Disorder who were hyperactive. She was just a natural teacher. I remember one day, maybe a week or two into the school year, she kept me inside one recess while the principal, Mrs. McLeod watched her kids outside.

"Don," she told me. "I know you have all kinds of energy. And that's good. But you know, when you are rocking back and forth it really bothers me and it bothers the other students too. In fact, any time you keep doing anything over and over and over again it bothers people. You know what I mean. Do you like the way Johnny M. keeps cracking his knuckles?"

I had to admit that I didn't even though I wished that I could crack my knuckles like Johnny could. And then she did a most amazing thing. She taught me how to keep doing something physical without bothering other people. Mrs. Carpenter had no training in how the left and right hemispheres of the brain work. She had no training in working with at-risk children. She was just a natural gifted teacher who had a child that was driving her nuts with rocking and had to do something about it. And so she did.

She told me that as long as I never did the same thing more than twice I'd be safe. "Three strikes and you're out!" was her motto. I could tug at my ear, but only twice in a row. I could even rock but only twice in a row and I had to complete at least twenty-five other motions before I rocked again! I could twiddle my thumbs. Twice. I could touch my nose. Twice. And on and on she went. She would do something physical like tapping a pencil. I would do it. During all the recess she had me sitting at my seat but always doing something different and never more than twice. Well, not exactly. Mrs. Carpenter knew that sometimes a person just has to keep doing the same thing over and over and over and over again. They didn't talk about perseveration[1] back then. Or how to treat it. She just did what she thought was right. She had me practice rolling my toes inside my shoes. Nobody can see that! And today I still sometimes move my toes inside my shoes when I feel that overwhelming urge to keep doing something.

What a gifted insightful teacher she was. She also made sure that no one made fun of me or Aaron Miller when we went to or returned from seeing the speech therapist. Actually, we might not have needed her protection. Aaron was the biggest kid in class. I was the toughest. Nobody messed with us. Nobody.

I never could quite match my brother Jack's academic achievements at Cook despite all the help I had from Betty June. He got all A's. I couldn't. I got A's in everything except, would you believe, handwriting. Here I am, the author of handwriting textbooks, and the best I could do was a C+ in handwriting all through grade school.

They had high standards at Cook School. Most people think that I have beautiful handwriting now. But I know better. Even though I might write a nicer script today than 95 out of a 100 adults, I'm sure I wouldn't receive anything higher than a C+ from my Cook School teachers if they were alive today to grade my handwriting. If it hadn't have been for Betty June and my great teachers, I probably would have been dysgraphic. Actually, I couldn't have been. They hadn't invented the term or concept yet.

The experts in dyslexia often point out that dyslexics tend to be artistic and musical. Well, in the 5th grade, I did win an art

---

[1]The word *perseveration* so loved by special education teachers is pronounced per SEV ur ray shun. It comes from persevere as in to persevere in doing the same thing over and over and over again.

scholarship. I got to go down to the Flint Institute of Art on Saturdays to learn how to mess around with clay. I wasn't impressed. I'd rather be playing football. I never did take all the free lessons. Some people think I'm an artist because I wear a Basque beret. More about that later. Some think that my illustrations for the book *The Tricky Words* demonstrate that I have artistic talent. Others have looked at my notes, which consist of at least 90% geometric doodling, and admire my artistry. I've been told by experts in the field of dyslexia that my doodling is a way to keep the right side of my brain from interfering with my left when I'm listening. To me, it's just a way to keep my body moving without resorting to rocking back and forth. An M. C. Esher, I'm not.

The school informed my parents that according to a test they administered to determine musical talent, that I was extremely talented and should be encouraged to learn how to play an instrument. Maybe they told all the kids that, I don't know. But I do remember taking the test which I thought was stupid. "Is this note higher or lower. How many beats do you hear?"

We had an old upright piano that had been given to us. About a third of the ivories were missing. Jack had taken lessons for a year. When he stopped practicing so did the lessons. Betty June had taken lessons for three years. The moment she stopped practicing, her lessons stopped. That was my mother's motto. No practice. No lessons. And don't ever think about asking for more lessons. One chance is all you get. I had two, maybe three piano lessons. But playing football was more fun. I wanted to *play* the piano, but I didn't want to practice. My mother said tough luck. No more lessons. But Betty June taught me some. She couldn't resist. Always the teacher. Today, I still love to *play* the piano. And I'm good enough to entertain myself. I don't worry about my mistakes. And I don't practice. I just have fun.

But there is something seriously dyslexic about it. As long as the sheet music has words, I can play it. I see only the melody line and the words. My right hand chords automatically. So does my left. And I don't know how. If the key the piece is written in is too high for me to sing along with it, I transpose it to a lower key. I don't know how I do it. I just do it. And sometimes when there's no one around, I'll take a book of ballads like those of Robert Service and put it up on the sheet music rack and create my own songs. What I call good poetry always generates a melody in my head and I just improvise. Again, I don't how or why. I just do. Maybe it goes back to the time when I was first exposed to language as a cranky baby. My family sang to me and danced with me. Words perhaps became identified with rhythm and melody somewhere in my brain.

Other things seemed to get lost in my brain, such as directions. Around our house Jack, Betty, and I had chores to do besides looking after baby Tom. Some chores were daily and some weekly. One of mine was carrying out the garbage. One night the whole family was seated around the kitchen table, and my dad asked me, "Don, have you taken out the garbage yet?" That wasn't a question asking for information. It was an order. I jumped up from the table, went out the back door, and picked up the garbage can. But, for some ungodly reason known only to dyslexic brains and absent minded professors, instead of taking the garbage can out to the curb, I brought it into the house. As I walked into the kitchen carrying it, nobody said a word. I walked through the kitchen, through the dining room, opened the door to the basement, and took the garbage can down into the basement and left it next to the furnace. Then I went back upstairs and sat back down at the kitchen table to finish my dessert. My dad just asked me, "Don, do you know what you just did?" I answered him, "Yes, I took out the garbage." He smiled and shook his head. But by then he was rather used to me doing strange things. "Uh, huh," he said, "And just where is the garbage now?"

It was only then that I could play back in my mind what had happened. I flew down the basement steps, retrieved the garbage can and took it to the curb. This is where I got one of my family nicknames, The Absent-Minded Professor.

The other nickname wasn't quite as friendly. It was Gypper. It resulted from my wanting to use a phrase that I had heard. I was playing checkers at the Cook School Summer Playground when an older boy thought he saw a good move for me. He asked to make the move. I let him. It resulted in my opponent being able to take a triple jump and get a king and take total command of the game. The older boy said, "I was gypped!" Actually, he wasn't. I was. But it made no difference, the moment I got home I had to find some excuse to use that word. At the dinner table I said, "Jack got a bike when he was ten. Betty June got a bike when she was ten. I never got a bike. I was gypped." And I never did. If I wanted to ride a bike I had to borrow either Betty's or Jack's. The nickname Gypper stuck. But there was a certain element of truth in my being gypped. At that time my parents were recovering from the blast of the Great Depression. "Waste not, want not" was their motto. Most of my clothes were hand-me-downs. Christmas and my birthday were the only times I got any new clothes. Christmas was always a time of great hopes and great letdowns for me. A pair of socks from dad. A pair of socks from mom. One set of underwear from Jack, one from Grandma. A book from Betty June. Maybe a winter shirt from somebody. That was it. Santa wasn't much better. The stockings were filled with walnuts, pecans, an orange, an apple, maybe a tangerine, and if I were lucky, one candy bar. I wanted toys. I kept asking Santa for guns, especially a B-B gun and a water pistol, toy soldiers, Lincoln logs, and an erector set. You would think that I would have lost my belief in Santa early when I never got what I wanted. But I didn't. I kept my belief long after my all my friends quit believing. I was stubborn. A trait some of my friends say I've never really lost.

But if I didn't get the toys and games I wanted at Christmas time, I did get what most kids never got. I got to play cards with the adults who came to visit. We didn't have television back then. So when people came to visit during the Christmas season, one or two card tables would be set up and the games would begin. Pedro was my favorite. But I loved to play Pitch and Smear, all three of which are variations on High, Low, Jack and the Game.

It never dawned on me that my parents were showing me off. I was their child prodigy at the card table. But for a dyslexic I can't imagine of a better preparation for winning at the game of life.

And I was good at winning at other things besides cards. Foot races. Wrestling. Football. Spelling bees even! I was used to winning. But there came a day that I misspelled one little word. I would remember that later on when I devised my Sequential Spelling. That was the day we had a spelling test on which occurred the word *shirt*. My teacher, like a great many other teachers, had each of us hand our paper to the person behind us to correct it as she read the correct spellings. When she got to the word *shirt*, the little girl behind me broke out in hysterical giggles. My teacher demanded to know what was so funny. The little girl told her! "Don spelled *shit* instead of *shirt*!" The class roared. The teacher tried to be stern, but couldn't help but laugh herself. Only one boy ever tried to tease me about it though. I pinned him quickly to the ground and pushed his face into the dirt. When I came to creating *Sequential Spelling*, I had ample data to back my concept that immediate student self-correction was the best method. Yet, I know that deep down my rationale was to prevent other little girls from laughing at other little boys just because they left the *r* out of *shirt*.

Cook School was where I got off to a good start. Had I gone to any other school in Flint, I probably wouldn't be able to read and write today. I probably would be in prison. I was no angel. And even though the statute of limitations has long since expired, I don't see any reason to confess now to the sins of my youth. I don't want to give my grandchildren any ideas. They have enough of their own.

Of the six kids my age that I played with in our neighborhood (East of Detroit St.), three ended up in Jackson Prison, one became a Catholic priest, another became a police chief, and the other a grocer.

Once in a while I played with my classmates who lived west of Detroit St. I loved their toys. I can remember Jimmy Murphy's toy soldiers and his erector set. And Timmy Patterson's Lincoln Logs. The other kids had toy guns. So we could play cops and robbers. But I couldn't invite them to my house. I was too ashamed. I was raggedy. I had no toys to speak of. Certainly no toy guns. I wasn't allowed to have guns or to play those nasty games such as cops and robbers. And I wasn't allowed to play in the street. And I didn't. Well, I didn't play in the street in front of our house, and I didn't play cops and robbers where I thought my mother could see me.

My older brother and sister knew. But they never squealed. They couldn't see what was wrong with playing in the street or playing cops and robbers. All the other kids did.

As well as I thought I was getting along at school, apparently some of my teachers recognized that I was different from the rest of the kids. They had me tested. I can remember going down for the psychological testing. It was a big game for me. I'm not sure what all the tests were about, but there were a lot of them. The upshot was that when the summer between fourth and fifth grade rolled around, I was enrolled in the University of Michigan's Fresh Air Camp. Lovely name. It was used to describe Cruickshank's camp for learning disabled and emotionally disturbed youngsters. It was the first such camp in the U.S.

All I knew is that I got to go to a camp. Most of my friends at school got to go to camps. Expensive camps. I thought I was finally one-up on my rich friends. I got to go to the University of Michigan's Fresh Air Camp and for a whole month! My mother later told me that one of the reasons I was sent there was because I had a compulsion to win. I never did like coming in second. Well, that's true. Maybe Grandpa Webb is to blame. He got me going early with knock rummy. Maybe I got hooked on winning. I don't know. All I know is that when I went to camp, I was the first to be assigned to a cabin. When the second kid came, I remember announcing to him that I was tough. I could beat up anybody in the cabin. The counselor was a bit nonplused. The other kid was twice my size. But there wasn't a fight. I talked tough. And that was enough. I never did have to fight at the camp. And I really had fun there. The only thing is, I didn't learn to swim. Looking back, I'm sure that this is somehow related to my learning disabilities, my dyslexia.

The year before my parents had sent me to take free lessons at the YMCA. I didn't learn. And I tried. I went to the Haskell Center for swimming lessons. They couldn't teach me. Maybe my skinny little body wasn't buoyant enough. I don't know. But I tried. And perhaps that's why I never accept an expert's opinion that little Johnny didn't learn to read because he never really tried. Trying is not enough. Just because the standard ways of teaching swimming may work for most kids, it doesn't mean it will work for all kids. Certainly, it didn't work for me. And more of the same still didn't work for me.

Not learning to swim even though I tried was my first real defeat. I stayed a red cap. White caps got to move into deeper water. Blue caps could dive into really deep water. My other defeat at camp came near the end. After the traditional telling by a counselor of the Hermit of the Lake story around the camp fire, and the big scare when the hermit appeared, we had a race back up the long hill to the cabins. There were about 150 of us. I came in second. And I remember being mad. Not angry. Mad. I felt I should have won.

The camp had very strict rules about parental visitation. Parents could not come to visit their children for two weeks. Mom and dad came on the first Sunday available for visiting. They planned a picnic for me. So into the family car they bundled me and whisked me off to a roadside park for the picnic. I gobbled down my food and asked them if they could take me back to the camp. I think I hurt their parental egos. I wasn't interested in seeing them. I was interested in having fun at camp.

World War II was going on at the time and my dad had a new job as the accountant for Kessel Tire. They now had enough money to rent a cottage for two weeks on Lake Lobdell. It was there that I learned to swim. But nobody taught me. I taught myself first to swim underwater with my eyes open and to pick up pretty stones on the bottom. Then I tried to swim regular free-style. I must have swallowed half of Lake Lobdell in the effort to learn. But learn I did. Grandma Webb always said that she was a stubborn Dutchman, and that's where I got my stubborn streak. And it was this stubbornness which those who admire me describe as persistence or tenacity that enabled me later in life to complete an analysis of the English language called *The Patterns of English Spelling.* More about that in Part 2, Chapter 12.

Starting in the third grade at Cook School we had a library class at least once a week. I can remember reading my way around the room. I started with the easy picture books, then the fairy tales, then the mythology. By the time I was in the fourth grade, I was reading the Tom Swift books and the adventure stories. What struck me then was that all of a sudden I went from books with lots of pictures and easy words to books with practically no pictures, long sentences and lots of big words. I couldn't understand then why there had to be such a big jump in difficulty levels. The question of why the jump in difficulty remained in the back of my mind for over forty years. It wasn't until fairly recently that I discovered why this sudden jump in reading difficulty in the fourth grade signals the end of reading improvement for so many students. My love of reading could very easily have stopped right there in the fourth grade, too.

It was sister Betty June who helped me overcome that big 4th grade hurdle. It also didn't hurt that my parents were talked into buying a set of encyclopedias called *The Book of Knowledge.* It was quite different from regular encyclopedias. It wasn't arranged in the customary alphabetical order. Instead, each volume had the same features, such as the "Book of Stories," "The Book of Things to Make and Things to Do," "The Book of History," and "The Book of Science." I started with just reading the stories. Then I dipped into the different sections. I don't recall ever using the set of encyclopedias for reference work. I just used it to read for enjoyment. The same with the companion volumes *Lands and Peoples* which was much like having ten years worth of *National Geographic* bound up into books. Among the other books that were around the house was a series of books about children from all different parts of the world. The titles always followed the pattern: *Little* _____ of _____ as in *Little Shawn of Ireland.* One book was about an Eskimo boy and how he lived. As a result of reading that book, I remember correcting my fifth grade teacher when she talked about Eskimos living in ice igloos. Remarkably, my teacher accepted my challenge and allowed me to bring my book to school and teach the class about the real type of dwelling they lived in during the winter.

Now, I understand how much I owe to luck, ignorance of my dyslexia by a loving family, the expectations of my parents, the expectations of my teachers in the best school in the city, and my sister Betty June. Without this particular fortuitous combination, I surely would be today just another one of the millions of functional illiterates in our society.

Chapter 3

Puberty, St. Mike's, diagramming and parsing

DESPITE THE FACT THAT I was the toughest kid at Cook School, I was probably the slowest in physical development. All the kids in my class had lost all their baby teeth and got their permanent teeth in before I lost my first tooth.

By the time I was ready to go into the seventh grade, my dad felt he could afford to take me out of the public school and send me to St. Michael's. I really wasn't prepared for 7th grade. But then, who is? It seemed that summer that all the kids my age grew at least three or four inches. I didn't. When I was in the 6th grade I was of average height. Or at least I thought I was. I was big enough to be the toughest kid in my class. No one beat me wrestling on the playground. I was captain of the 6th grade softball team. I remember hurling a no-hitter. I won the 50 yard dash and the broad jump. So I couldn't have been too much below average. But in the 7th grade and at a new school suddenly I was the smallest.

But I still *thought* I was the toughest kid. That is, until I got mad at John Ford. I was going to beat up John. Now, John stood about six foot and weighed close to 200 pounds. I was almost four foot ten and weighed maybe 70 pounds. John just picked me up off the ground and held me in a bear hug. The best I could do with my arms pinned close to his chest was to try to pound on his chest and scream, "Let me down, I wanna beat you up!" John just laughed and laughed and laughed and held me until I finally came to my senses.

My stay at St. Michael's taught me a number of different things. One, it taught me all about diagramming and parsing. Oh, I really enjoyed that. For the rest of the kids who had always attended St.

Mike's, it was the same old thing that they had been doing for years. For me, it was new and exciting. Diagramming was logical. It made visual sense to me. And I'm glad I went there instead of continuing in the public schools because the Flint Public Schools had thrown out diagramming and parsing. They were into something new in English. I'm not sure what they called it then. But whatever it was, it didn't help the students learn much about our English language.

One thing I didn't learn anything about *at* St. Michael's was sex. My entire formal sex education was limited to a statement by my mother that I shouldn't be worried if some morning I woke up and I was wet but it wasn't pee. And if I never do, I shouldn't be worried either. I understood the warning about wet dreams or nocturnal emissions. I had already experienced them. My informal sex education was quite a different story. The University of the Gutter gave me all kinds of wild and incorrect ideas about sex. At St. Mike's not only did we have a class clown, we had a class pervert.

I learned more than where babies came from while I was at St. Mike's. I also learned a bit about prejudice. Not racial prejudice. St. Michael's parish was the Irish parish. Names like Purcell, Donovan, Goggins, O'Connor, McCabe were the rule. Very few Negroes in Flint were Catholics. The few who were Catholic belonged to Fr. DuKette's parish which was so small it had masses only on Sunday. To supplement his income, Fr. DuKette often said the 6:00 mass on Saturday at St. Mike's. I liked to serve mass for him. He didn't waste any time. Only Fr. Ceru could whip through the Latin faster than Fr. DuKette. Race and racial differences just didn't come up in class or outside of class, at least not around me. It never occurred to me that there might be anything wrong with different types of people living in different neighborhoods. I never encountered any of the systematic training to hate other people as in the song from *South Pacific*, "You have to be carefully taught before you are six or seven or eight to hate all the people your relatives hate. You have to be carefully taught."

My first experience with prejudice had nothing to do with race. When my parents began to notice that I was squinting a great deal, they took me to an optometrist. Sure enough, I needed glasses. Now, not only was I the shortest kid in my class, I was "Spec's." The nickname was not an affectionate one. I was an Altar boy and sang in the choir. That helped. But I never was invited to the other kids' parties. I was an outsider. But I felt I could make it into the inner circle if I were able to demonstrate my athletic ability. So in the spring of my ninth grade I went out for two different things, forensics and the high school baseball team. Forensics, I made. I won a dictionary for winning the district in extemporaneous speaking. For baseball I had the same coach, but that was a different story.

It was a cold, wet spring. So cold and so wet that the coach Tom Smith could have only one day for tryouts. His idea of a tryout was to line everybody up by height and count off 1-2-1-2-1-2. The 1's went to bat. The 2's went to the field. I played second base and never made an error. At the plate I scraped up a walk and three singles. I stole second base twice. I would have stolen second four times except that twice there was a teammate standing there. Remember my friend Aaron Miller who went to speech class with me at Cook? Well, he struck out every time at bat. But he made the team, and I didn't. True, he was six foot one and two hundred pounds and his foul balls were out of sight. Tom Smith could see his potential. Me? I was so small and scrawny he couldn't see any reason to put me on the team even though I was perhaps the best infielder, the best hitter for singles, with my almost microscopic strike zone the most likely to get walked, and the fastest base runner. That did it for me. No way was I going to return to St. Michael's in the fall. And I didn't.

Chapter 4

Flint Tech–a high school without a gym.

INSTEAD OF RETURNING TO St. Michaels, I went to Flint Technical High School. It was a different kind of school. It had no gym. It had no library. It had no cafeteria. It had no auditorium. It didn't even have a single foreign language class—not even Latin. And yet, this school, was by far the best high school in Genesee County.

Flint Tech was really a creation of General Motors with a good deal of help from Citizens Bank and other members of the Flint Chamber of Commerce. GM supplied the equipment for the machine shop. Tech supplied graduates who went into the skilled trades for GM. The businesses in Flint provided part time jobs in the afternoon for the co-op students.

Flint Tech had the best high school teachers. The only weak teachers were the football, baseball, and basketball coaches, all two of them. But that's not why I chose to go to Flint Tech. I chose to go there because it was the closest high school to where I lived. I could walk there. And besides, my brother Jack had graduated from there. To be painfully honest about it, I think the real reason I went to Flint Tech was that Flint Tech was the arch rival of St. Mike's in football and basketball. If I couldn't play ball for St. Mike's, I'd play against them.

I didn't know that to go to Tech every student had to have at least a 3.0 average in junior high and to stay there had to maintain at least a 2.5! But what a difference it made. At Flint Tech they had good discipline, good students, and good teachers. We didn't have to worry about drugs or guns or violence. In fact, I was perhaps the biggest trouble maker for the teachers in my class.

I enjoyed baiting teachers. My favorite stunt was to look out the window while the teacher was talking and to pay attention.

Inevitably, the teacher would try to make an example out of me. The teacher would call on me fully expecting me to say "What?" And then she could tell me to pay attention. Only it never worked that way. I would answer the question without bothering to turn my head! More than once the teacher was so furious that I could look out the window and still answer the question that I was sent down to Mr. Mehring's office.

In the spring of my tenth grade at Flint Tech, I tried to go out for Forensics and baseball again. This time, forensics was out. The school had dropped it. But I did go out for baseball. And this time, I made the J.V. team. In one game, I stole nine bases: second base three times, third twice, and home four times. Of course, I was stealing off the pitcher. His coach hadn't taught him how to properly take a stretch. He would pull both hands back which is a wind up and then he went into a stretch. By the time he threw the ball I would be standing on the next base.

Did I get congratulated by my coach? Was my feat ever recognized? No. In fact, the coach was furious. You see, he wasn't there for the game! And he had left strict orders that no one was to steal without being given the sign. And every base I stole (which was every one available to me) was without a sign. I was told I would have to sit the bench for the rest of the season.

In high school I was into all kinds of things. I was on the student council. I was on the Junior Town Hall of the Air. I became president of the Hi-Y (a YMCA organization for high school boys). And I got a job at Herrick's Drug Store. Most of my jobs were custodial such as sweeping the floor, burning the papers, stocking the cigarettes, wrapping up the Kotex and Modess. In those days, women never bought Kotex from a man, and certainly did not want anybody to know what it was she was buying. And condoms were hidden away in drawer out of sight where generally only the pharmacist on duty would be. These, I didn't stock. But I knew where they were. I had seen the owner open that drawer and fish out the Trojans and the Sheiks. I even knew that sometimes they were referred to as rubbers or three-for-fifties. But the words *condom* and *prophylactics* were not in my vocabulary. As I said before, my sex education was conducted in the University of the Gutter. That's how things were back in the 40's. One day when the pharmacist was out eating his supper a man came into the store. The fact that he walked by Shirley and Joan and came straight toward me should have been a clue. But it wasn't. Dyslexics aren't always that fast on picking up on things like that. Clue number two was that he *whispered* to me, *"I'd like some prophylactics."* But all I heard was the word *prophylactic* and I had seen it someplace. Yes, on some toothbrushes. But I was new. I couldn't remember where the toothbrushes were. So, I turned to Joan and in my normal loud voice said, *"JOAN, WHERE ARE THE PROPHYLACTICS?"*

The man's face turned beet red. So did Joan's face. Finally, it dawned on me what he wanted. "Oh, you want some Trojans not toothbrushes?"

It was working at the drugstore that enabled me to grow up and be cool. I could learn to smoke while burning the papers in the alley behind the drugstore. Oh, what I went through just to be able to be cool. But I wasn't about to smoke in public as a kiddy-puffer. I was going to be cool. I would be able to inhale and hold it and then let it out slowly. I would be able to blow smoke rings. But first I had to be able to stand up! The first puffs made me dizzy. But I was stubborn. Just like learning to swim, I was flat out stubborn. I kept coating my lungs with tar until I could inhale without getting dizzy.

My dad didn't like it. My mother didn't like it. But grandma secretly shared that vice and whenever mom was out of the house, the two of us would sit around and smoke and talk. My dad said smoking would stunt my growth. Sure. As if my growth hadn't already been stunted. Mom said it was a sin. Yet, she couldn't explain why all the priests at St. Michael's smoked.

Just like I had believed in the advertising about Santa Claus and believed in Santa Claus long after my classmates had become skeptics, I believed in the cigarette advertising. Cigarettes are for the mature, for the cool. The leading men in the movies always had a cigarette. Heroes smoked. And so would I.

In my junior year, I made sure we had forensics. I lined up a teacher to be the sponsor. I went from homeroom to homeroom explaining what forensics were and recruiting students to try out for it. My efforts paid off. We ended up with a good team. I decided to try out for Oratory and help coach someone else in extemporaneous speech. The coach, Helen Massey, helped the other students with their declamations and dramatic declamations.

1948 and 1949 was a time of communist conspiracy hysteria. My oration was timely. It was: "Wake up America before it's too late!" It started with those words and ended with those words. In between I was almost a junior Joseph McCarthy. The difference was only that I was quoting from magazine articles out of *Time, Newsweek,* and *U.S. News and World Reports.* I wasn't making things up. I was repeating as gospel things that Joseph McCarthy and those of his ilk had made up and had been dutifully reported by the news magazines of the day.

I now am a little more skeptical about what I read in the newspapers and magazines than what I was then. Just as I am a little skeptical about "out-of-body" experiences that I hear reported. The reason? My oratory evoked one. I had an out-of-body experience caused perhaps by stress and full knowledge of failure.

What had happened was that I had won the district in oratory and now was in the regionals. The night before the contest, I attended one of our basketball games. McCabe, the one man cheering section, cheered the team on to victory. When I woke up the next morning, I could barely talk. And I had to compete in oratory!

I went. I was determined to win despite my laryngitis. When we got there, I was horrified. The contest was being held in a regular classroom. No stage. No audience. Just judges seated in the front row. I started with my "Wake up America before it's too late" and the next thing I knew I was watching myself and hearing myself delivering a flat monotonous speech. Needless to say, I didn't win.

Even though I had never played tennis before, I went out for the tennis team. Chutzpah, for sure. Believe it or not, I made the team. Dyslexics sometimes do the strangest things. Just as Tech didn't have a gym, didn't have a football field, or a track, it also didn't have a tennis court. We practiced at Flint's Ballenger Park. It was only two and half miles away. Nobody had cars at school. To get there by bus would have required bussing downtown and then transferring. By bus it was at least an hour away. We could walk it in a half hour. And we did.

I wasn't a star. The only reason I made the team was that so few went out for it, that all I had to do was to beat out two klutzes for a spot. But I do remember one great victory playing doubles. We were playing Flint Central (one of the state's better tennis teams) at our home court, Ballenger Park. Keith Emerick and I were partners. We served first. I never could hit a hard serve, so I used a cut serve which came as a surprise, I suppose, to my opponent. He hit it high and way out. Knowing Ballenger, I knew where that ball would go if I let it bounce. It would go up and over the fence. So I stepped back about three steps behind the base line and caught the ball. "Our point! Our point!" screamed our opponents. "You have to let it hit!" We gave them the point. They were right. Those are the rules. But, oh, what a controlled adrenaline flow it gave me. I never stroked the ball so hard and so straight at opponents as I did that game. They knew I was trying to hit them. And I was! And I did! And Keith and I were the only Flint Tech players to win a match against Central. It's amazing how brain chemistry can work. There's no way Keith and I should have won. Our opponents were clearly much better than we were. But controlled anger will beat fear every day of the week. We were angry. They experienced the fear of getting hurt. Fear of losing. Fear. Later on I was to incorporate the concept of eliminating fear of failure into my method of teaching spelling to dyslexics.

During my senior year, my brother Jack who had graduated from Tech married Thomasina Barone, a St. Michael's graduate. Their marriage took place on the same day that Tech and St. Mike's had their annual football game. What a day that was! I was one of the altar boys and I watched my Uncle Ted, who was best man, do something absolutely unforgettable. The wedding ring had been tied to a little pillow so that the ring bearer wouldn't lose it. When the pillow with the ring was handed to the priest, the priest couldn't untie it. But no problem. Uncle Ted just reached into his pocket and pulled out an unwrapped double-edged razor blade. The priest's eyes just popped. The wedding was in the morning and the reception followed soon thereafter. It was at Brookwood Golf Club. It was a festive Irish-Italian wedding. The booze was flowing. That day no one said a word about my drinking except my sister Betty June.

"Don," she said, "Every time I see you, you have a different drink in your hand. You'll get sick doing that." I didn't. Just like I started to become a skeptic about cigarettes, I was beginning to be skeptical about the myths surrounding drinking.

My dad wasn't concerned about my drinking. Social drinking was part of our family life. I was a senior in high school, and it was time that I joined the adult family. All he said to me before the reception was, "Don, don't you dare drink so much that you embarrass the family." Later on, he told me he was disappointed in my behavior at the reception.

He said, "Don, every time I saw you, you had a cigarette either in your hand or dangling from your mouth."

He didn't mention anything about my drinking. I didn't stay until the end of the reception. I had a big football game to attend. I almost was thrown out before I got in. The ticket taker could smell the alcohol on my breath when I was about ten people back in line. When I got up there to get my ticket, I recognized the ticket taker. He was my math teacher. He looked at me, shook his head, and warned me about getting into trouble. I didn't. Not that night anyway.

The next week in student council I did get in trouble. The assistant principal came in and abruptly announced that the senior class would not be able to have their annual winter Snow Ball. That really upset me. I snapped angrily at him, "But we reserved that date way back in February. You can't do this to us."

"Oh, yes I can," Mr. Mehring said. "And there's nothing you or I can do about it. It's just a matter of priorities and commitments. There are only so many Friday nights available for dances and we can't have dances when we have home games or games that are in town. We have promised the holders of Student Union cards five dances. Right now there are only four. The only night available for the fifth student union dance is the night that the seniors have planned to have the Senior Snow Ball. Sorry, but that's the way it has to be."

I was not easily turned away. Dyslexics can sometimes be as stubborn as bulldogs. And sometimes just as vicious.

I then said to him in a very cold hard tone bordering on sarcasm, "I notice you didn't say anything about Saturday nights."

His answer was the school couldn't have a student union dance on a Saturday night. There's no way they could get teachers to chaperone.

"That's a lie!" I said to him. "I already know of two teachers who said they would be available to chaperone." And as president of the Hi-Y, I wasn't bluffing. During a Hi-Y meeting we had discussed the possibility of a special Saturday night dance to raise money for Bruce Jepson, a football player who broke his leg in a game and whose family didn't have any medical insurance to cover his bills.

"And besides," I said, "there's no reason why we can't have parents as chaperones. I know my parents would chaperone a student union dance. And I'll bet most of the parents on this council would chaperone if asked."

Mr. Mehring sputtered, "Well, I don't care how many teachers or how many parents you can get as chaperones for a Saturday night student union dance, we just can't possibly have a school dance on the eve of a religious holy day like Sunday."

"Mr. Mehring," I said in even colder and harder tones just dripping with vicious sarcasm, "Just what kind of a religious bigot are you? You're willing to have dances on Fridays, the eve of the religious holy day of Jews and Seventh Day Adventists, and not on Saturdays?"

What I said was not kind. The way I said it was absolutely cruel—but effective. Mr. Mehring stormed out of the room.

Fifteen minutes later he came back with the principal, Mr. Olsen. Mr. Olsen assured the student council that something could be worked out. The Senior Snow Ball would be held as scheduled.

Mr. Mehring never forgave me. And even though I ended up graduating 2nd in a class of 174, I never was inducted into the Tau Sigma, the national honor society. Any faculty member could blackball any applicant. I suspect Mehring did that to get even with me. But it could have been almost any of my teachers. I was far from the model student.

Tech was a small school and class schedules weren't very flexible. In my senior year, I went on co-op working in my father's accounting office in the afternoon. Unfortunately, the only time trigonometry was offered was in the afternoon. As my lowest grade in math at that point was an A, I felt I could take the class without going to class and pressed my point with the principal. Little did I know at the time that I was putting the principal on the spot. I didn't know that he was a golfing buddy of my dad's. I didn't know that he kept my dad informed about my progress in school. I didn't know then that it was my dad's friendship with the principal that got me into Tech in the first place. It also allowed me to be the only student in the school that was neither on a technical curriculum or a business curriculum, the only two that were offered. I was taking courses from both curricula so that I had basically a college prep curriculum minus the language requirement but with business and technical courses thrown in.

A conference with the trig teacher was arranged. As long as I did every homework problem in the book and handed in the homework before I left for co-op and as long as I could maintain at least a B average on my tests for which I would have to go to class, he would allow it.

So I quickly formed an alliance in study hall with five other trig students to study together. We would divide up the problems six ways and do them. We didn't just copy from one another. We taught one another. The proof of our ability to work together and teach each other was demonstrated on the tests. The six of us were the only ones to get A's on all the tests. This experience was really the basis for how I taught a class called Modern Grammar years later. See Part 3, Chapter 11.

So I spent my afternoons working for my father in his office in the Mott Foundation Building. At that time, my dad shared an office with an automotive parts sales firm that was owned by Harry Eiferle who also was the manager of the Mott Foundation Building. Probably because it was convenient for Eiferle, my dad's office was right across the hall from the office of Charles Stewart Mott. He was the largest single stockholder in General Motors and was a well known philanthropist. C. S. Mott was also quite a character. He always wore an old fedora, a wrinkled suit, and carried a battered old brief case. He had his own grass tennis court and loved to play tennis in his bare feet. And he always had a smile for me when I passed him in the hall or rode in the elevator with him. He knew me by name. And I'm sure that if he would have lived long enough, like to the age of 130, he would certainly have seen to it that the AVKO Educational Research Foundation which I started would have received a large start-up grant from his foundation. But at least I got to know personally one of Flint's best known and best loved personalities when I was a senior in high school.

I didn't belong to any of the cliques. But I did have two very close friends. One was my tennis partner Keith Emerick, a Protestant, and Mason Himelhoch, a Jew. We were sort of three musketeers of a different sort. Keith went to the University of Michigan and majored in atomic physics. The year 1950 was a bad time for doing that. I believe he ended up being exposed to far too much radiation and he died before he was thirty from cancer. I don't know what became of Mason. And I suppose he doesn't know what became of me. But that's the way it goes after high school is over and everyone goes his own way.

Chapter 5

Junior College–chess, bridge, and pinochle.

DESPITE THE FACT THAT I had won a full-ride scholarship to the University of Chicago, my parents wouldn't hear of me going to that hotbed of atheism. Especially after my cousin Bob McCabe had gone there. It didn't matter to my folks that he was successful. What mattered was that he didn't believe in God. At that time Bob was working in Washington. Later on, Champagne Bob (as J. P. McCarthy calls him) eventually became the president of Detroit Renaissance and was well known and respected in the highest of circles in Detroit. But I wasn't to be allowed to go to the University of Chicago. My parents were afraid that in that hotbed of atheism I would lose my religion.

So, I went to Flint Junior College for two years instead. There I enjoyed the freedom of being able to cut classes. And cut them I did. I played cards in the men's union from eight in the morning until 4:30 in the afternoon. I took occasional breaks for classes. I learned how to play bridge and pinochle. Chess I didn't master. I learned how the pieces moved. I learned the rules. But I just didn't really understand the game. All I knew is that I hated to be humiliated, and there was a student there who enjoyed whipping his opponents at chess. He spotted me a bishop and beat me. He spotted me a bishop and a knight and beat me. He spotted me a queen and beat me. Then he spotted me all his pawns and still beat me. Damn! I didn't touch a chess board again until I got to the University of Detroit.

When I wasn't playing cards in the Men's Union, I was in the office of *The College Clamor*, the student newspaper. I covered the games for the sports section and eventually became the sports editor. The paper's faculty advisor was Charles Donnelly. He had also been (as I had found out later) the faculty advisor for the Newman Club. This was a Catholic student organization that was present on almost every public college campus in the United States, except ours. Here it had been banned. I hadn't realized how much anti-Catholic sentiment existed in Flint until then. Later on, I was to discover that at that time there was an unofficial quota for both Catholics and Jews in the Flint School District. But the fact that it was banned didn't really bother me. I just helped revitalize the banned organization. In the process I found out who had been president when it was a legal student organization, a student by the name of John Means. I would later meet him at the University of Detroit.

I tried to get the Newman Club's activities mentioned in *The College Clamor*, but everything I wrote was censored. I tried writing letters to the editor. They were censored. I tried to write an editorial about the situation. It was censored. Then I went to the Clamor's business manager Ann Smith (who would later become my wife) and bought an ad for a Newman Club dance to be held at St. Michael's Father Murphy Hall. That was censored.

I stormed into the office of the president of Flint Junior College and demanded an explanation. He hid behind a weird interpretation of the U.S. Constitution. "It would violate the principle of separation of church and state." The fact that the type of censorship the Newman Club was faced with amounted to a denial of freedom of speech did not impress him.

Neither was he impressed when a week later I brought to him petitions signed by two hundred students asking for the formation of a Phalanx Club, a coed non-denominational organization affiliated with the YMCA and YWCA.

The year was 1951. Demonstrations on college campuses were unheard of then. In the sixties they would be commonplace. We almost had one. The students were upset when I told them that not only couldn't we have a Newman Club, we couldn't even have a Phalanx Club. There was to be an assembly for something or other the next day. Ten of my friends told me they would make up picket signs and march around the auditorium and totally disrupt the assembly. We planned a real doozy of a demonstration. But all I could think of was how my dad would react. He would crucify me.

I called it off. I said to my friends, what my Grandpa Webb always told me. "You can't win a pissing battle with skunks. We won't get the Newman Club going. We don't have the money for an attorney. And if the YMCA won't take them to court, what's the point? So shuffle the cards and deal."

In one way, I wish I hadn't called it off. But now I know, if I wouldn't have called off the demonstration, I would never have gotten my top secret security clearance that enabled me to go into the Army Security Agency. The FBI and the CIA took a dim view of protesters and trouble-makers. As it was, it seemed as if everybody who knew me was interviewed. Years later I would find that out in talking with friends, neighbors, and business acquaintances of my father. But I got my clearance and was able to get in the Army Security Agency. It was there that I had a number of experiences that eventually would enable me, a dyslexic, to really crack the code of the English language in such a way that I could discover a way to help other dyslexics learn the code.

But at the time I had no idea that I would be in this area. But I did know that my father would have been embarrassed by a college demonstation led by his son. He had connections in the community. This my sister Betty June was thankful for. Because that year she had graduated summa cum laude from Marygrove College and with a teacher shortage on, she thought she would have no problem getting hired by the Flint Schools. She couldn't believe it when her application was turned down. She was in tears. My dad asked her if she would mind terribly if he made one telephone call on her behalf. She reluctantly agreed. Dad called Frank Manley and explained the situation. Frank, being a Catholic, knew what had happened. The Flint Public Schools had already reached their quota of Catholics and Jews. But Frank headed up the Mott Foundation. He was the one that developed the concept of the Community Schools that eventually spread across the country into just about every school system in the United States. Frank made one phone call. Ten minutes after Dad made his phone call, the phone rang. It was someone from the personnel department of the Flint Public Schools wanting Betty June to come down and re-apply. An opening had just occurred. Amazing.

AN AUTHOR'S INTERLUDE:

Today, I was reminded rather forcefully of just how dyslexic I still am. On the telephone I had to take down the name of a person. It was a Ms. Heather Pottle. But I couldn't hear Pottle. I heard "Toddle." And I just knew that wasn't a good name. So I asked for the spelling. P as in Peter and then all I heard was ? ee ?ee EL ee. Three times I had to ask. And I'm not hard of hearing. Never have been. But it's always been easy for my mind to play games with what it hears. A few hours later I was working on this autobiography and I wrote, My brother older Jack instead of my older brother Jack. Then coming home with my wife from the Clio Golf Club after dinner, I happened to remember that our daughter-in-law had called earlier in the day and had asked for her. It took me two full minutes to come up with her name. My wife even gave me a huge hint saying, "Remember what you said about why she named her first child Jason?" I kept using all my normal methods of recovering words and names of people I know by using associations. Eventually I came up with Joan by linking it with Bob and _____. It was only then that I remembered how I had jokingly said after their first child was born that they found a unique way of naming their child after both of them. Jason Robert is an anagram of Joan's Robert. Yes, I am dyslexic and always will be. And sometimes it's even fun. Frustrating, but fun if you can learn to laugh as hard at yourself as I laugh at myself, sometimes.

Back to Junior College: chess, bridge, and pinochle

That my mind had been developing a little differently than normal people's minds do, is illustrated by an incident that occurred in my *Introduction to Psychology* class. At the beginning of a class that I actually attended, my instructor announced he was going to conduct a little experiment. He drew a line on the chalk board. He asked us to take out a piece of paper, put our names on it, and then estimate the length of the line he drew. He collected the papers and then asked us to read in our books while he compiled our answers. He sat at his desk for about ten minutes ostensibly tabulating our answers while most of us read. Then he passed back our papers. He then stated that the average guess was 40.37 inches for the line. He asked us to then look at the line and estimate one more time, and to be sure to put the second estimate directly below the first.

That direction was wasted on me. I didn't change mine. I saw a yard stick lying on the chalk rail. The line was about two inches longer than the yard stick. I stuck with my 38 inches.

It didn't take the instructor long to analyze the results. Everybody whose first estimate was more than 40 inches lowered their estimate. Everybody whose first estimate was less than 40 inches raised theirs. Everybody, that is, except me. The instructor used the experiment to explain the phenomenon of subtle peer pressure. He also said, "Apparently, Mr. McCabe, has a very independent mind. He's the only one I've ever had in this class who didn't change his mind when I've conducted this experiment."

Maybe *independent* is another word for *stubborn*. Whatever you call this trait, it certainly applies to me. It manifested itself in many different ways. One was when I was at one of the underground Newman Club dances held at Fr. Murphy's Hall. Mike Burke and I went there together in hopes of picking up a couple of girls. While we were there we spotted two girls dancing together who looked rather sharp. So, we naturally tried to cut in. Lo, and behold, they said almost in unison, "No, thanks. We'd rather dance with ourselves." Mike and I were dumbfounded. Just then, the Mexican Hat Dance started. Mike and I looked at each other. We didn't say a word. We just started dancing the Mexican Hat Dance. We put on such a display that everybody stopped dancing and formed a circle around us. The two girls who wouldn't dance with us, didn't get to dance that dance. When it finished, Mike and I were given a thunderous ovation. Men never danced with men, but we did that one time.

No other girls refused to dance with us that night. We had a ball.

At that time part of the requirements for a college degree demanded that we have eight hours of science. Even though I had straight A's in chemistry and physics in high school, I couldn't see any point in taking more of the same. Geology was a subject that qualified as a science. Even though it was taught by a known task-master who never smiled, Lynn DuPree, I took it. He didn't scare me. After all, DuPree was the moderator of the Bridge Club and had taught me to play bridge using the Culbertson system.

There was something about his grading system that I admired. Something that I hadn't seen before or since. He announced to his class that there was never any point in arguing about a grade on a paper or a test. He didn't care if he made a mistake that would change your grade. Don't hassle him. He didn't average grades. He believed that if you were an A student you would get mostly A's. Three A's and one E in most classes would average out to a B. But not for him. Whatever was the most common grade was your grade. Mostly B's you got a B. Mostly C's you got a C.

The first semester went by quickly. He had multiple guess tests. And at multiple guess I always was good. I had no grade lower than A. The second semester I started with an A on the first test. Then Mr. DuPree got sick. A substitute was brought in. Ugh. She was bad. She lectured in a monotone that would put an insomniac to sleep. When she gave us her first test, it was an essay test with one question: Define evolution.

I thought that was easy enough. I thought I understood Darwin's theories from beginning to end. And away I wrote and wrote and wrote. I covered everything from natural selection to genetic mutations induced by chemicals, exposure to ultra-violet rays, etc.

When I got the test paper back, it had a big E scrawled across it with the comment, "You didn't use the words _**sudden change**_." That was it. The only time I returned to that classroom was with Mike Burke to booby trap her desk with a live mouse we had caught in _The College Clamor_ office.

A month later DuPree was back. The first thing he did was to give us a test to see what we had learned in his absence. I had the lowest score in the class. But it really didn't matter because nobody passed. He gave us a stern warning and then proceeded to begin from the beginning and put it to us.

The next test I got an A. On all the subsequent tests through to the final I got A's. Mr. DuPree called me in to his office one day and said, "McCabe, I hate you. I have never had a student like you before. And I know I won't ever again because I only have about a month to live. You have nothing but E's and A's in my grade book. More E's than A's because I was out so long. I can't flunk you. I wish I could, but I can't. And I don't care if you did score the highest on the final exam, I'm not going to reward you with an A. All I can do is give you a C. Now get out of here."

Part of the graduation requirements was that I would have to take a speech class. I fought it. Why should I take a class in public speaking when I already could speak in public? I showed them my record. I had won awards in both extemporaneous speaking and oratory in high school. It still didn't matter to them. I had to take some class in public speaking. They would allow me to take Debate and have it count. Debate was a fun class even though I had to compete against Willy Barker. He was a Cook School kid that I never had to beat up. He didn't play sports. He didn't play on the playground. He was what today we might call a nerd or a geek. But I would rather compete against him than with him. I thought I had a great partner even though my partner was a she, Wanda Burkes. At that time, I didn't think much about girls having the intelligence to make a good debater. I did make an exception for my sister, Betty June. She was bright, but she was an exception. Wanda proved a great complement to my style. I was the firebrand. I was the attacker. She was the quiet soft spoken half of the team that gave it balance. I didn't realize it at the time, but our team was probably the first racially mixed debate team in the state of Michigan.

When my parents saw a picture of our debate team, and saw that Wanda and I were partners, they never said a word. But then again, they had never said anything about my running around with Keith Emerick, the Protestant, and Mason Himelhoch, the Jew.

It wasn't that I was a liberal. I was just naïve. I didn't know what white society thought I was supposed to know about Negroes. Dyslexics often are naïve. They don't pick up on subtle prejudices. It needs to be hammered home. I hadn't really been exposed to racial prejudices or stereotyping. My racial naïveté would, however, bring the wrath of my dad down on me, but not until after I graduated from college. And that was not because he felt I had no right to have Negroes as friends. No, it was because I had unwittingly put my life and the lives of two other people in jeopardy by "integrating" an area dominated by the Ku Klux Klan.

Chapter 6

University of Detroit, Ph.B.=Piled Higher and Better.

I DIDN'T ATTEND THE graduation ceremonies at J.C. where I was awarded an Associates in Arts degree. That was just a break between my sophomore and junior year as far as I was concerned. But that break was slightly interesting. That was the one summer I spent as a counselor at the Mott Camp working with the boys the Flint Schools thought could benefit the most from the experience of camping.

It was fun. It was frustrating. And I learned a bit about how naïve little boys can be. For example, we counselors played guessing games with them. One was to guess our ages. The boys in my group unanimously agreed that I had to be at least forty years old because I had such hairy legs.

I also exhibited some trust in my instincts. There was a boy who just stood around holding a Bible in his hand who wouldn't participate in the activities. He would just stand stiffly. Or sit stiffly. That wasn't right. The very first opportunity I had I went to the camp director, a psychology major, to tell him about the kid I suspected to be practically a catatonic schizophrenic. He laughed at my suggestion. "If he were, he'd be in an institution, not at camp." But, he begrudgingly agreed to look at him. When he did, he called social services and saw to it that the boy would begin to have some therapy. He told me later that he couldn't believe that the boy was sent to this camp. The kid needed heavy psychiatric treatment.

When I got down to the University of Detroit, a Catholic university run by the Jesuits, it didn't take me long to get involved in the St. Francis Club. It was something like a Greek fraternity, except that we were bonded together somewhat differently. We were a group of out-of-towners who banded together to have a place where we could have good food and not have to pay through the nose for it. We were all depression babies that were going to college. This co-op was what we needed to survive.

I also got a job working in the office of The Student Counselor, Fr. Foley. It was there that I demonstrated graphically the dyslexic's ability to lose all sense of time. One of my jobs was to alphabetize all the class cards of all the students at U of D. 1952 was a long time before computers! After my eight o'clock French class on Mondays, I had a break until 1:00 when I had English Literature 201. So I started working on those class cards for Fr. Foley. At about 11:30 I looked at my watch and decided I would work for another half hour and then go to lunch. Every so often I would look at my watch and see that it was 11:30, decide I would work for another half hour and then go to lunch. I probably did that about twenty times or so. Then Fr. Foley stuck his head out of his office, and said, "Don, it's after five. I don't pay overtime. See you tomorrow."

Since I had no idea of what I wanted to do after I got out of college, I was enrolled in a liberal arts course that led to a Ph.B. degree. There are very few of us who hold that degree. And I'm proud of it. Those of you who have a B.S. degree know what B.S. stands for and it's not brown sugar. M.S. stands for More of the Same. Ph.D. is just Piled Higher and Deeper. My Ph.B. is Piled Higher and Better.

The moment I got into the St. Francis Club, I tried to get my roommate Jaime[1] Persivale to join the St. Francis Club, but he wasn't interested. He didn't need it to save money. He was from Lima, Peru. He came from a wealthy family. He also was the leader of the Latin and South American students on campus. Our room was a meeting place for them. It was inevitable that I would learn some Spanish, mostly that which I would never write in a book like this.

---

[1]The name Jaime is pronounced "Hi, me." Some people have Americanized the name so that it is pronounced "Jay me."

Jaime was a real athlete. If U of D had had a soccer team, Jaime would have been on it. He was a star back home. I saw some of the pictures he had in his scrap book I also watched him dribble a ping pong ball on the toe of his foot! He was good. I only played ping pong once against him. He beat me not with one hand tied behind his back but by hitting the ball behind his back! Whew!

The hardest part of making it through the pledge period at the St. Francis Club was in getting to know each member's name and where they were from. Names have a way of slipping out on me. When a member asked you something you had to somehow use their name and where they were from in your answer. Often I had to come up with other information about them, such as their year in school or the course they were on, their girl friend's name or whatever before I would finally get it. Maybe I made it because they enjoyed watching my agonizing. Or maybe it was because the president of the club, Alex Zukowski, loved to play bridge and I was always available to be the fourth.

As you can imagine the training by my grandfather in card playing helped me master the game of bridge. Well, at least to a stage above where the rest of the players were. Having learned Culbertson, I now turned to Goren and quickly memorized the Goren bidding system.

It just so happened that the best chess player at U. of D. was a member of the St. Francis Club. He also wanted to learn how to play bridge. He asked me if I would teach him. Dyslexics can be opportunists. I agreed on one condition, and that is, he had to teach me how to play chess. He didn't have to teach me any rules or how to move the pieces. I already knew that. I also knew that there was something I had to learn but what it was I didn't know.

That little something was how to look at a chess board. What to look for. What type of overall strategy had to be used to be a winner. Things like that. Like my grandfather, he too, was a good teacher. Before long I was giving him real battles and then finally our battles were so equal, we might as well have flipped a coin before we started to declare the winner.

We never kept track of who won the most games, and I'm glad we didn't. That way we both can feel that we won a few more than the other.

Author's interlude #2

In a re-reading of the manuscript I asked my wife if I should include a certain incident that occurred in my Adolescent Psychology class. I thought it might help the reader to understand how dyslexic minds not only tend to be extremely logical but also tend to reject the illogical. Blind acceptance is not typical of dyslexics. Independence is. My dyslexic in residence, Philip B., who also had read the manuscript, said it was just another one of my rebellions. Is that another example of a dyslexic automatically not accepting and seeking another explanation?

I'll leave it up to you to judge. My Adolescent Psychology class was taught by an instructor who was a Hungarian refugee. His accent was thick. His knowledge of American customs was meager. His concept of testing and evaluation flat out stunk. Can you imagine a class in which the final grade was based on only two tests, the midterm and the final? Sure you can. But can you imagine this as the midterm exam?

Directions for Midterm Exam: Choose either but not both parts. Part I. List the stages of development NOT according to your textbook but as per MY notes. Part II. List ten adolescent psychology textbooks and their authors.

I wrote my name on a sheet of paper and the following sentence: *This is not a test. This is an insult.*

I stormed from the back of the room up to his desk. I slapped my "test" paper on his desk and repeated for all the class to hear, "This is not a test. This is an insult."

When I left the room I was followed by at least a dozen students. But my chutzpa didn't end there. I visited his office and challenged him to have any of his A students compete against me on an objective examination prepared by any other psychology teacher. "Flunk me and I promise that the president of university will hear about your asinine testing and grading system." He gave me a C.

End of Author's interlude #2

Two of my closest friends at U of D were Paul Klozik and John Means. Paul had been a star basketball player in high school. In the army he was assigned to special services to play basketball. Unfortunately for Paul, his team lost in double overtime in an army tournament. The winners stayed stateside. The losers went to Korea. Paul was hit in the knee with shrapnel and taken prisoner. Although he received some medical attention from the Chinese doctors, it came too late. They saved his leg, but he would never be able to bend it again.

John Means was also a Korean Vet. When I met him, he was surprised to know that I knew he had been president of the Newman Club at J.C. John also happened to be a Black. But the color of his skin meant nothing to Paul nor to me. It was John's wit that mattered. He wasn't a comic. But he was sharp. He was analytical. He was a good conversationalist. He also was a good drinker, meaning that his demeanor never changed no matter how much or how long he drank. He always was in control.

So when graduation time came, I wanted to have one last fling with my close buddies. I knew I wasn't going to get any graduation gifts. My dad felt helping pay for my tuition to U of D was gift enough. No more was needed. So, I did manage to swindle my father into giving me a different type of graduation gift. I asked my dad if I could have John Means and Paul Klozik up to the cottage for the first week after graduation. He agreed and so it came to pass that the three of us had one last blast together. We had fun. We went canoeing down the Rifle River. We golfed at the West Branch Country Club. We had cook-outs. We went to the resort area bars and restaurants. And that was in the year 1954 when, as I was to find out later, you rarely saw a Negro north of Bay City.

But we weren't interested in integrating Northern Michigan. We weren't civil rights advocates. We were friends.

When the last day of our stay, Saturday rolled around, my family came up. Nobody blinked. John and Paul were introduced. Dad seemed to enjoy talking with them and arguing politics with John. My dad was a staunch Republican. John, a Democrat. Paul and I were independents who would argue either side of any issue.

When Paul and John left, my dad lit into me. Not in front of my younger brother Tom and my younger sisters Mary and Nan. He waited until they went down to the beach, and then, wham! He lowered the boom. He let me know in no uncertain terms I had no business risking the lives of Paul and John nor risking *his* property. He explained very emphatically that every time a Negro bought a cabin in this area, it was bombed out. Over and over he stressed just how stupid I was to risk their lives and his property by bringing a Negro into an area ruled by a very active Ku Klux Klan.

Part II – Twists and turns of fate that prepared and led a dyslexic into teaching dyslexics and finding out what dyslexia is all about:

Part I dealt with my education from birth through college.

Part II covers the period in which my real education began. It will also explain why the materials and techniques I developed to teach dyslexics could not possibly be developed in a traditional academic method.

Part III covers the techniques and materials that I developed because of my own dyslexic symptoms and outlook, techniques and materials that work. If you're already convinced I know what I'm talking about, you could skip Part II. But I'm prejudiced. I think Part III will make more sense when you know exactly where I'm coming from and where I've been.

Chapter 7

The ASA: Learning Russian in California and Teaching English in Japan

WHEN I GRADUATED from the University of Detroit, I didn't want to go job hunting. In 1954 most employers didn't want to hire anyone who was draft bait. My college deferment was over. So rather than wait around, I volunteered for the draft.

Because the soonest they would take me was in November, I took a grounds maintenance job working for Joe Szilagyi at Brookwood Golf Club. He made sure I was in top physical shape for the basic training.

Perhaps it was the fact I was in better physical shape and a few years older than most of the men, that convinced the barracks sergeant to make me a platoon leader. I was gung-ho. Now one of the first things that happened was that we all took a battery of intelligence and aptitude tests. On one of them I scored high enough to be tapped by the Army Security Agency. They wanted me. And the ASA had first choice.

But the results of the tests were not given out until nearly the end of basic training, just before the bivouac. Apparently the barracks sergeant saw the results. Instead of being a physically hardened hardnosed private that would make a good platoon leader, I was just one of those egg-heads who were going to go into the the Army Security Agency.

So all of a sudden, I was relieved of my responsibilities of being platoon leader. Then, on the first night of bivouac I caught guard duty. One night without sleep isn't so bad. I handled the next day's activities with no real problem. Then I was assigned guard duty again. It was supposedly a random thing. It was harder to stay awake this time, but I was in top shape. I could do it. And do it, I did. The third night, they selected guard duty a different way. And again, I had guard duty. That wasn't a coincidence. That morning we packed up our gear and started to march the 15 miles back to our barracks. I started out somewhere near the back of the main group. It was one of those hurry up and wait marches. Well, I was exhausted physically, mentally, and emotionally. I wasn't going to run to play catch up and then stand and wait. I walked a comfortable pace. Rather quickly there were two groups of men. Those in front and those who couldn't keep up who brought up the rear. I was marching to my own drummer somewhere between the two groups. With the Company Commander looking on from his jeep, my barracks sergeant ordered me to either join the first group or fall back with the second group.

I told him to go to hell. He started toward me. I threatened to kill him. I raised my M-1 to an attack position. I used a few very typical army expletives and let him know very clearly that I wasn't going to let him continue "messing" with me. He backed off. I marched by myself between the two groups back to the barracks. I had fully expected to be called into the CO's office. I wasn't. I didn't say anything to the other men. And the other men didn't ask me any questions. Basic training was over.

After a short leave I reported to Ft. Devens to sit around waiting for my Top Secret Security Clearance to come through.

Now, anybody who has been in the service will tell you never volunteer for anything. And they're right with one exception. Back then not many men could type and I knew the army ran on typewriters. Today, it's computers, but back then it was typewriters. At the very first morning roll call after arriving there, the sergeant asked if anyone could type. I volunteered. The next thing I knew I was working for the 1st Sergeant and making out the duty roster and typing out the weekend passes. Guess who never went on K.P. and who always had a weekend pass! All of us there had to wait until our clearances came through before we could go to an ASA school. I quickly found out what school I would be going to. It would be the Morse Code school. The thought of spending eight hours a day listening to and transcribing dit dot dits was not at all appealing to me.

When I found out that the ASA was also looking for candidates for the Army Language School, I asked to take the test to see if I could qualify. Test taking had become a game to me. It was a game I was good at. I passed with flying colors. Now, I had to extend my tour of duty if I wanted to go there. I figured one more year would be worth it. I'm sure I was right.

My Top Secret Security Clearance was slow in coming through. Of my group from Ft. Leonard Wood, I was one of the last to get mine. That's why I am so sure that if I would have allowed the protest demonstration to take place at Junior College, either the FBI or the CIA would have refused to grant my TOP SECRET clearance.

The day after my clearance came through, I was sent to the Army Language School in Monterey, California. Once there I had to learn Russian and in a hurry. The army did have a very strong motivational device. Pass and you automatically have a PFC stripe. Flunk and you go to Korea in the infantry. That's real carrot and stick motivation.

Very few ever flunked. First of all they used good screening devices. The average I.Q. was more than one standard deviation above the norm. The language aptitude test took care of the rest. But even then, it's a good thing the Army didn't do what most publishers do. They didn't call up a name university and ask to have the resident "expert" develop the teaching materials. They also didn't go to the universities and ask for teachers who had been certified by the State of California to teach. No, they wanted native speakers for their teachers. These native speakers developed their own texts. And they used teaching techniques they were familiar with. These are techniques that were not then and still are not today used in American schools to any real extent at any level.

Learning Russian was the first real academic challenge I faced. I had to learn a new language and fast and compete against students who not only were bright but who were not dyslexics like myself. Of course, at that time, I didn't even know what the words *dyslexia* and *dyslexic* meant. All I knew is that compared to the others there, I had problems learning. But I learned.

And I learned from teachers who wouldn't be allowed to teach in any American public school. Why? Because they had not been taught how to teach by teachers who don't know how to teach. You know the old saying: Those who can, do; those who can't, teach. Well, it's been my experience that those who can't teach, teach the teachers. More about that later on.

What I learned at the Army Language School was that the teaching of phonics works, especially in such a phonetically regular language as Russian. We learned to write the alphabet which has a few letters that are just like ours such as the letters a ("ah") and o ("oh"). But some Russian letters just look like ours, such as the Russian *P* which corresponds to the English *R* and the Russian *П* which corresponds to our *p*. And then we have the funny looking: **ж, б, ю, Ё, ф, и, ш, л, д, ь, щ, й, ы, г, ц, ч,** and **я**.

Everything at the Army Language School was carefully structured. Direct instruction was employed in small teacher controlled classes. The part of the direct instruction that helped me more than any other part was the dictation. Sentences spoken at normal conversational speed had to be written down correctly. The hardest part for me was to determine where one word stopped and another started. One phrase in particular stands out in my memory because I mangled it so completely:

"*NAH•BARE•UH•GOO•WRECK•KEY.*"

I had no idea how many words were in the phrase. In fact, because it was spoken so fast I couldn't repeat in my head those six syllables. Not until my instructor helped me to break it down into *NAH* plus *BARE•UH•GOO* and then *WRECK•KEY* could I even repeat the phrase after her. Then and only then could I translate it as "On the river bank." Literally: "On bank river's"

I now know where part of my problem was. The moment I have any unknown sound of more than three syllables, it blows right by me. And I'm sure that same phenomenon occurs even with many non-dyslexics, for all intensive purposes. Yes, I know it should be "for all intents and purposes" but that *is* the way I heard that phrase for about the first forty years of my life.

Every hour we had a different teacher. They were up front about the reason. They wanted us to learn to react properly to differences in the dialects used by these native speakers. They didn't try to teach us just one correct dialect. They wanted us to be able to translate into proper written Russian the words no matter how slurred or accented by dialect. If I had not been exposed to this method of teaching at the Army Language School, I'm sure I would never have been able to design AVKO's "Spoken Dialect Translation Exercises" or to come up with the concept of "SCRUNCHED UP" speech.

Another aspect of the effect of "grammar" and "intonation" within language was lodged permanently in my memory for over twenty-years before I fully understood what it was all about.

Because our teachers were native speakers of Russian, they were still learning to speak English themselves. Book English they knew. The common idioms of spoken language and the slang of the streets they didn't know. And they wanted to learn it. So they very often traded "language secrets" with us. In exchange for learning the *#@! words of English, they taught us the Russian equivalents. Off the record, of course.

One day on a smoke break between classes two students were flipping and matching quarters. Our instructor whose nickname was Honey Buns asked them what they were doing. Not knowing her intent, one of them responded, "We're jess flippin' quarters."

When the bell rang to start the class Honey Buns, eager to use her newly acquired slang phrase, asked the class, "Anyone want to flop me for a nickel?"

━━━━━━━━━━━━━━━━━━━

Nobody volunteered. We just doubled up in hysterical laughter! What she said could really only be interpreted by native speakers of the American language as soliciting. Cut rate or major discount, it could only be soliciting. Even though we all knew it couldn't possibly be her intent.

After we had finished the crash course in Russian and just before we were shipped back to Ft. Devens, we were treated to a weapons display at nearby Ft. Ord. We saw all kinds of weapons, Russian, Chinese, British, Japanese. We were allowed to touch them, to hold them, to familiarize ourselves with them. Finally we came to this one rifle that I happened to pick up. I could hardly believe how heavy and clumsy it was. It was then that I was almost killed by the Master Sergeant guide who thought I was being a wise ass. All I did was ask a simple question, "What's this?" The rifle was the M-1. The same one I had with me all through basic training. The same one I had to be able to take apart blindfolded and put back together. In less than a year I had forgotten something I had been using every day for six weeks.

I didn't understand it then. I do understand it better now. Six weeks of intensive learning is not necessarily enough to lock knowledge into a dyslexic's mind. I know because I worked with one dyslexic intensively for six weeks. He lived, ate, slept, and studied at the AVKO Reading Clinic. His reading level soared from the 4th grade level to the 9th grade level. His reading speed on easy reading went from 40 words per minute up to 120 words per minute. When he returned home to Texas, I gave his parents a detailed prescription on how to continue the AVKO program at home. Unfortunately, his parents failed to incorporate the tutoring program into their busy daily routines. Within six months all his gains had been lost just like my knowledge of the M-1 had been lost. With dyslexics the "use it or lose it" concept really applies.

My next stop was the Voice Intercept School at Ft. Devens. It was hush-hush. We weren't supposed to tell anybody anything about what we were studying. Top Secret. Here we studied how to work with short-wave radios, tape recorders, and tell the difference between commercial Russian radio traffic and military Russian radio traffic.

We weren't allowed to take anything into or out of the building where we studied. The competition was intense. One student sneaked some material out to study. He was caught, court-martialed, and given a dishonorable discharge. So much for the study ethic.

Our class was told that half of us would be sent to Europe and half to Japan. Whoever scored the highest would get first choice. Whoever scored second highest would get second choice, and so on until all the Europe or Japan choices were taken. Those on the bottom would have no choice.

The way the school determined passing or failing was by an arbitrary score of let's say 750 points out of a possible 1,000. I don't remember exactly. But I did know that I had already posted forty more points than the minimum for passing. All a perfect 100% would do for me would raise my passing score. I had already passed. I didn't know which choice would have been better for me. We weren't told where in Europe we would be assigned. We knew nothing about the working conditions of the different types of jobs our training had prepared us for. So I did what many dyslexics might do. Nothing. I put my name on the test answer sheet with the comment. "I've already passed this course. I don't care to compete over where I'm going."

So, for the first time in my life, I graduated from a school dead last. My assignment: Japan. Looking back on my rather bizarre behavior, I now realize something else might have been operating in the background. I had just quit smoking cold turkey. At that point I was smoking a pack and a half a day. The way and the why of my quitting smoking is a little peculiar but revealing. I woke up one morning during my last week of school at Ft. Devens, sat up in bed, reached for a cigarette and then started my hacking and coughing up a bit of phlegm. A thought flashed through my head: *I really ought to quit.* Then another contradictory thought hit me: *I can't quit. I just bought two cartons of cigarettes and a new cigarette lighter*!

If that last thought makes sense to you, then you don't understand how logical most dyslexics are. I suddenly became angry at myself for being so terribly illogical. **Quitting** smoking was logical. That hideous, insidious and perverted rationalization of saving money by continuing to smoke got to me. I was so angry with myself for even allowing that irrational thought to enter my mind, I immediately gave away both cartons of cigarettes and my lighter.

About the only thing relating to dyslexia that took place on the troop ship to Japan had to do with seasickness and the concept of *expectations*. Nearly every soldier on board got seasick. They expected to. And they did. There were only fourteen of us specially assigned Army Security Agency personnel on board. We all knew that seasickness had to be more psychological than anything else and we weren't going to get sick. Well, one of us wasn't so sure. He brought along and took his Dramamine. He used drugs. Thirteen of us decided to enjoy the rocking motion and have a positive outlook. It worked. Only once did I come close to vomiting. That was in chow line. The private behind me puked over my shoulder and filled my tray with his vomit. The cooks were understanding. They allowed me to get a new tray and start through the chow line again.

The fourteen of us went to a processing camp outside of Yokohama. From there we were to be assigned. The ASA headquarters in Tokyo got first choice. So I didn't go there. The ASA base in Hokkaido, the Japanese version of Siberia, got second choice. So I didn't go there either. The bottom of the class is the last to be picked.

I got stuck with being stationed just outside the only city in Japan to be spared in World War II, Kyoto, the most beautiful city in Japan. How lucky can a dyslexic graduating at the bottom of his class get!

The next two years were undoubtedly the most enjoyable years of my life. At our base our section worked twenty-four hours a day. To do this we had four shifts but only three working on any one day. For example, my shift might start working six days (8 AM to 4 PM) and then get two days off. Then we would work six days (4 PM to 12 Midnight) and then get two days off. Then we would work six days (Midnight to 8 AM) and then have another two days off before repeating the cycle. But because my section was so overstaffed we usually had two days off each six working days. That amounted to four days of work and four days off. So when I took leaves I only took four day leaves on the four days I was scheduled to work. If I timed my leave just right, I could get 12 consecutive days off for the price of just four days of leave time. And I used up all my leave time while in Japan!

For the first time in my life I kept a journal. So many things were happening around me. And for the first time in my life I really began to educate myself. Up until this point, I hadn't really been close to any truly educated and intelligent people. There is a difference. Despite my Ph.B. and my majors in literature and philosophy at U. of D, I was out of my league. Some of my best buddies would in casual conversations drop names such as John Dewey, Alfred North Whitehead, Immanuel Kant, and Bertrand Russell, just as easily as basketball fans can drop names like Charles Barkley, Magic Johnson, Michael Jordan, Shaquille O'Neal, and Isiah Thomas.

When I wasn't working, playing chess or bridge, teaching English to Japanese English teachers at the American Cultural Center, visiting the bars, or playing the tourist, I was reading. Never before or since have I read so many books. Never before or since was I so determined to build my vocabulary, to make sure I could understand everything someone was talking about, to make sure I could understand what I was reading. I hadn't realized until then that I had been in the habit of just blipping over words that I really didn't know and not really knowing that I didn't know them.

I can't emphasize enough the importance of knowing what it is you don't know.

> If you don't know that you don't know,
>
> you can't begin to learn.

This, I'm afraid, is the case of all the biggest names in education today. They know a great deal. They're not dumb. They're well educated. They keep up with each other's work. ***But they don't know what it is that they should know***. Anybody's work that is outside their own closed circle, the big names choose to ignore. For example, why should they read this book? They already know all they need to know about dyslexia and teaching children to read. They won't read it unless they are paid to review it. At a book exhibit, they walk right by. Nose in the air. If they don't stop, if they don't look, and if they don't ask questions, they don't run the risk of letting people know that there might possibly be something they don't know.

So many things happened to me while I was in Japan, that I could (and did) write a book about them.

Remember how I quit smoking? Cold turkey. Strong stubborn streak. But I liked to smoke. I liked to be sociable. The Japanese loved American cigarettes. So dumb me, after a year without a cigarette, thought I could smoke sociably. Uh huh. And the Pope is a Baptist who likes to hunt penguins in the Sahara. Sure. So, I started carrying cigarettes with me. They were only 15¢ a pack back then. I could afford that. And sure enough, I got hooked again. It didn't take me long to start smoking two to three packs a day. A man of moderation in all things. Uh huh.

But not only did I learn history, literature, and philosophy by reading when I was in Japan, I also got the opportunity to study Russian. After about a year, one department euphemistically called Traffic Analysis needed an extra body. Our Voice Intercept was still overstaffed. And I was the lowest on seniority so I got transferred. What I saw was an incredible waste of time and money. Everybody in that section drank coffee, smoked cigarettes, wandered from desk to desk with papers in their hands, and shot the shit. By three o'clock they had an hour to go, and they got their work done. Everybody was ready to go at 4:00. I was shown what I had to do. After I mastered the intricacies of the job, I decided enough was enough. I wanted out and back to my Voice Intercept job with my friends. What I did was simple. I did my work. I did my work in forty-five minutes. Then, I sat at my desk studying my Russian. There wasn't much they could do. I got called on the carpet, of course. The officer in charge of the section accused me of reading instead of working. I corrected him. I said I was studying. The subject I was studying was my primary Military Occupational Specialty (MOS). I told him I should be commended for my ability to do my work and for improving my MOS skills by studying instead of wasting time with frivolous conversation, as the others in the section were doing. He didn't like my attitude at all. I wasn't a team player. He threatened to assign me to a different daily traffic analysis report. I told him fine. I could handle that. I told him there wasn't a job in the traffic analysis section that would take me over an hour to complete.

He sputtered, fumed, and dismissed me. He must have known that he was in somewhat of a bind. He could have tried to have me face some kind of kangaroo court-martial. But he also knew I was his superior officer's favorite duplicate bridge partner. I played duplicate bridge with the C.O. at the Officer's Club at Camp Otsu. Because I always wore civilian clothes and because officers weren't supposed to fraternize with enlisted men, I was always introduced as being a civilian from the National Security Agency (NSA) staff that was on our base.

I don't know if the solution to the problem was his, a group decision, or the commander's decision. At any rate, I was sent back to my regular section on the pretext I was incompetent. For them to have properly made use of me, I would have to attend a special school. So by being supercompetent where I didn't want to work, I got kicked back to where I wanted to be. I wonder if Professor Peter would have approved?

Being a volunteer teaching English in English to Japanese college students and Japanese teachers of English was an incredible experience. Twice a week I went down to the American Cultural Center and taught. I made a number of good friends and learned a great deal about Japanese culture and traditions. I also learned that when English is taught as a second language by someone whose native tongue is not English, the students rarely learn to understand spoken English. It took me a while to figure it out. Basically it's the same reason why so many American students misspell the following phrases:

Correct spelling:	Typical misspelling
supposed to	sposta
used to	usta
have to	hafta
should have	should of
what did you	what you (whud juh)

When teaching English in English to Japanese English teachers and college students, I spoke in my normal American speech patterns and rhythms. I DID NOT SPEAK SLOW LEE AN'Duh CARE FULL LEE EEE NUN SEE ATE EACH WORD. Instead, I just spoke normally. This they wanted. They wanted to be able to understand Americans when they spoke.

But very often I would have to translate. For example, one day I started class by saying in my normal fast but sloppy mid-western speech,

"Whudduhyuh wanna cover today?"

I got blank stares. So I wrote it out on the board: What do you want to cover today?

I underlined What do you and said "Whudduhyuh." Then I broke it down "What" is slurred into "whuh" and "do" is slurred into "duh" and "you" becomes "yuh." *Whudduhyuh* means *What do you.* *Want to* becomes *wanna.* They all knew the meaning of the word *cover.* But they didn't want to put something on top of another thing. They wanted to learn English. So I "covered" the idiom *cover.*

Another time a student was puzzled by the word *affection.* It didn't make any sense in the sentence to him. So I started to explain what *affection* meant.

"No! No! It can't mean that!" said one of the teachers of English from Doshisho University. "Affection means disease."

I quietly but firmly contradicted him with "I think you're confusing the word *affection* with the word *infection.*" .

Out came the pocket dictionaries. The whole class was gibbering away in Japanese. And then one after another they tried to point out to me that I was wrong. Unfortunately, I couldn't read Japanese. I had to take their word for it that their dictionaries defined *affection* as *disease*.

Knowing I was right, I simply stated that even dictionaries can make mistakes. This they couldn't accept. So, away to the huge unabridged *American Heritage Dictionary of the English Language* I flew.

I read and explained the definitions. But then I saw an entry that blew away my mind. There *is* a medical definition. Affection *does* mean disease! That part of the body *affected* by the disease is the *affection*!

All I could tell them was that the writer of their pocket sized English/Japanese dictionary must have picked what he thought was the most logical definition and ignored all the others. As a result he happened to hit upon a definition used only by the medical profession. Even then, most doctors and nurses of my acquaintance told me that they had forgotten that medical definition of *affection* when I told them this story.

Later on I was to draw upon these experiences in Japan to develop a method of teaching American students how to translate their speech, their "Ah wanna's," "Ah gotcha's," "Yor gonna's," "We hafta's," and "He sposta's" into the correct written English equivalents of "I want to...," "I got you...," "You are (or You're) going to...," "We have to...," and "He is (or He's) supposed to..."

I will never forget those two incredible years in Japan when I learned more about the Russian language and especially my own English language then I ever did in school.

Chapter 8

Time out to write a novel and get married.

I RECEIVED MY DISCHARGE from the army in December 1957. Waiting for me at Bishop International Airport in Flint was my fiancée, Ann Smith. We didn't rush into a marriage. We had known each other since 1950 when we were both on the staff of *The College Clamor* at Flint Junior College. But before I settled down, I just had to try my hand at writing a novel based on my experiences in the ASA.

So for about a year or so I pounded away on an old electric typewriter. The title? *8610 Topeka.* The cast? Members of the Army Post 8610 that worked in the section whose TOP SECRET code name was Topeka. It wouldn't be right to reveal the plot, but it did contain some scenes that the CIA and the FBI probably did not appreciate. For example, did you know that in 1956 there was an American base that went out on strike? Yep. You guessed it. Our base went out on strike. It never hit the papers, the radio, or TV. But we had a strike. Technically, it was a mutiny. But we preferred to call it a temporary work flow stoppage caused by equipment failure. The problems with the equipment were only solved after an order from Tokyo putting a curfew on our base was rescinded and all the privates were promoted to PFC.

Years later, when I ran into some former members of the ASA who had served in other parts of the world, I found out that our strike wasn't unique. Other ASA bases had been hit with strikes. None, however, were ever reported in the media. What has that to do with my novel? Maybe nothing. Then again, maybe everything. From what I understand about the publishing houses, is that when a book comes in over the transom as they call it, it goes through a slush pile. The bottom rung "editors" glance at them and send out polite rejection notices to at least nine out of ten that are given to them. If by chance one looks halfway interesting to them, it goes to another reader a little higher up on the ladder. He automatically rejects nine out of ten of these. The one out of ten that gets through the second stage (which is now one out of the original 100) goes to a third reader. That takes time. But usually it doesn't take four months for a book to be rejected. Each time mine was rejected, it took five months.

Why? I don't know. I suspect that key parts of my novel were sent to the CIA for their approval. With the U.S. deep in the Cold War with Russia, it wouldn't surprise me if the CIA told the publishers that our National Security could be jeopardized if the book were to be published.

Only a few people ever read the manuscript. Perhaps someday I'll return to it. I think it was a damn good book. But then again, I'm prejudiced.

After finishing my novel, I had to go to work. My savings were exhausted. I checked out the want-ads. There were very few job openings anywhere. I answered an ad that sounded promising. When I went I listened to a beautiful spiel. What they wanted me to do was to place *free* (?) sets of *Colliers Encyclopedias* in homes as part of a grass roots advertising campaign. All the people had to do to receive the free set of encyclopedias was to listen to the full explanation of the program and then promise to keep them up to date by purchasing once a year for only ten years a book that updated the set. Easy money, guaranteed. All I had to do was knock on doors and place sets and the commissions would roll in. Well, I tried it. I knocked on doors and swindled people into buying the encyclopedias. I tried to convince myself that because the *Colliers Encyclopedia* was such a good product, that the sales pitch was just that, a sales pitch. I did that for about two months, outlasting the staff who were there when I started. But I didn't make a killing. I didn't really make a living.

Just barely enough to get by on. When I fast-talked a minister into accepting a "free" set of encyclopedias even though I saw that he already owned two other sets of encyclopedias, my conscience finally got to me. I quit.

I heard from a friend that National Cash Register was hiring. So I applied for a job with NCR. I took their placement test and scored way too high on it. So high that the man who interviewed me hesitated to hire me. He told me that I might be a bit too bright to be a cash register salesman. But I did answer his first key question correctly. He asked me, "Do you believe people are basically honest?" I answered, "No." He asked me why and what I told him was almost word for word the big sales pitch of National Cash Register. That is, if a person has both a need for money and the opportunity to steal it, the person will. Need and opportunity are the sales points for NCR. Since everybody has some need for money (real, imagined, or psychological) the best way to keep employees from stealing is to limit the opportunity and NCR's cash registers were the answers to every retailer's dream.

That may have been, but it wasn't for me. To be a good salesman you have to handle rejection. It was the old theory, knock on enough doors and someone will buy.

———

I married Ann Smith on December 7th, 1958. We had met at Flint Junior College. She was the business manager of the College Clamor. I was the sports editor. We had dated at J.C. and off and on while she went to Michigan State and I to the University of Detroit. When I was in the army we became engaged. And that created a few problems. She was a Protestant. I had been born and raised a Roman Catholic. And interfaith marriages were a big no-no back then.

Ann took instructions and was willing to raise our children as Catholics. But something funny happened on the way to the altar. This something which wasn't really funny took place while I was in the army. I've already said that during the Army I did more reading than at any other time in my life. What I didn't say is that I also studied other religions and other philosophies. When I was in Japan I took three separate administrative leaves that by definition didn't count against regular leave time. One was to take a Catholic retreat. One was to take a Protestant Retreat. One was to take a Jewish retreat. If I would have had the opportunity for a Buddhist or Moslem retreat, I'm sure I would have taken them as well.

Now, back home, I was no longer absolutely positive that the Pope is infallible. I no longer believed that just because I was baptized Catholic and had the sacrament of Confirmation when I was twelve, that I was bound for life by the laws of the Catholic Church. It's not that I wanted to leave the church. In fact, I tried to get priests to convince me that my reasoning was faulty. I was very curtly and rudely rejected by four different priests. They didn't have the time to "save my soul." If I wanted to save my own soul, I would just have to believe. "It's just a matter of faith."

It's also a matter of record that I no longer attend church. Whether I'm better or worse for attempting to practice the major beliefs of all religions seven days a week instead of just once a week, I leave to God to decide. So be it.

I could no longer accept the church's doctrine of the infallibility of the Pope. I had lost my faith in organized religions. So I couldn't in good conscience have a big church wedding inside St. Michaels church. I couldn't very well have a big wedding in Ann's church. My family and their friends would not have attended. And they had told me that. Even my sister Betty June had tried to talk Ann out of marrying me. And for many years all my family followed the party line of Roman Catholicism and refused to recognize our marriage. No congratulations were given. And not a single wedding present. Why? Because to them, I was living in sin. I was the black sheep. To say one nice word or give a present could be construed as condoning sin. They stopped counting the months on their fingers after a year had passed and we were still childless.

Ann's parents were a bit more accepting—once they realized I wasn't going to force Ann to convert or to force her to agree to raising our children as Catholics. They even came to our little wedding on Sunday, December 7, 1958. Her sister Marijean and Marijean's husband Charles Kroell were witnesses. Bill and Beverly Rue were guests. And that was it. Well, not quite it. I should admit that I never did recite my vows. Dyslexics do have a problem repeating things. And I never did get it right. After about four tries, the minister just skipped over my part and continued on with the ceremony and eventually pronounced us man and wife. I often wonder why we weren't pronounced woman and husband, woman and man, man and woman, or wife and husband. Language is strange. So maybe Ann and I aren't married after all. Maybe we're just lovers who have stayed together and raised a family of our own.

We never did have a honeymoon. Ann went to work the next day. I went back to the University of Detroit to take my education classes that would enable me to become certified to teach school.

Although not one member of my family recognized our marriage at the time, most of them recognized it by the time our twenty-fifth wedding anniversary rolled around. We got a lot of lovely cards. Does that sound like I'm bitter? Well, maybe I am a little. But I still love them all. They're family. And other than my marriage to Ann, they have been there for me when I needed it.

Part II, Chapter 9

Teacher certification: A time consuming farce.

WHEN I WAS IN SCHOOL, teachers were my opponents, my enemy, all except my sister Betty June. I never knew what I was going to be, but I just knew I would *never* be a teacher.

At various times I had thought about going into law or medicine or the priesthood. When I discussed my plans for the future with my parents, they flat out said I should never become a lawyer because I was too honest and had too strong a sense of right and wrong. To be a successful lawyer, my parents claimed, you had to be without a moral sense. They didn't think medicine would be a good field for me either. They felt my feelings for people were too strong. They believed that because I had such an apparent need to win and not lose, losing my patients to the grim reaper would hurt much more than simply losing my patience with a client. As far as being a priest was concerned, they thought I might make a good one but that I should wait until I was at least twenty-five before thinking about going to a seminary.

My dad had wanted me to be an accountant like himself. He gave me great training in his office. How great? Great enough to allow me to skip Accounting I, II, and III in college and to go straight to Accounting IV, Cost Accounting. But I didn't want to follow in my dad's footsteps. Besides, my older brother Jack was already positioned to take over my father's accounting business if and when my father ever retired. Working for a father is tough enough. Working for a father and an older brother would have been too much for me and much too much for them.

So with my wife supporting me, I went back to school to take enough courses in Education to get my teacher certification. That was the absolute worst academic experience I ever had. How bad was it?

Bad, bad, bad. It seems that there is a great deal of truth in the old saw: Those who can, do. Those who can't, teach. Well, those who can't teach, teach the teachers. For those of you who are teachers, you already understand, or should understand. For those of you who went to college and took subject matter courses, it may seem difficult for you to understand just how bad teachers of education courses are.

In my Methods of Teaching English class I was told that there are two ways of grading compositions: A single grade and two grades; one for content and one for form. Wow! I was impressed. I had to take a class to learn this?! The text was perhaps as bad as the teacher.

One of the tests I took should illustrate the vapidity of the courses. You see, I took a test in a course I wasn't taking. I still feel rather embarrassed by the whole episode. I had two different 4:30 classes, one on Mondays and Wednesdays and the other on Tuesdays and Thursdays—both in the same building! As you know many dyslexics have a tendency not to know what time of day it is or *what* day it is. One afternoon I was playing bridge at the St. Francis Club and suddenly realized that was 4:35. I was already late for class. I rushed across Livernois Avenue dodging traffic, ran to the Arts and Science Building, and tried to slip into the class quietly. Someone was sitting in my seat. It hadn't dawned on me that I went to the wrong classroom. Oh, well. This is college. Everybody was busy taking a test. My instructor walked over to me and handed me a test. I went to the back of the room and sat down and took the test.

The next week my instructor said to me, "McCabe, you gave me a terrible start last night. I had just finished checking all those tests and was putting the grades in my grade book. Your name wasn't there. I thought I was losing my mind until I realized you weren't taking my Education Through the Ages class. You're in my Educational Psychology class instead."

What embarrassed me the most is that as I was taking the test, I didn't realize that it was in a subject I wasn't taking nor had I ever taken. And I aced it! Strange! To me this episode rather epitomizes college education classes. Mickey Mouse.

Part II, Chapter 10

Teaching the bright. Baby sitting the others.

THERE WAS A TEACHER shortage back in 1959. I had no problem finding a job. But the first job I was offered was unbelievable. My certification was for high school English and any subject at all in junior high. I was offered a job teaching grade school with the assurance that I would become a principal as soon as I could get the appropriate elementary education classes. The salary and the promise of rapid advancement in a growing school system was attractive, but I felt certain that I wouldn't be able to live with my conscience if I accepted it.

I did interview for a job with the Flint school system. I was offered a job teaching English and French in a junior high. I told the man interviewing me that I didn't mind teaching in an inner city junior high, but I could not in good conscience teach French. Russian, yes. Latin, maybe. French, No. My college classes in French were bad. There were no language laboratories. There had been no effort to teach us to pronounce French correctly. Since two years of a foreign language were required for a liberal arts degree, the teachers of those language courses hated to keep a student from graduating just because they were not proficient in the language. I freely admitted that I had bluffed my way through the tests. I freely admitted that I really couldn't speak or read French well enough to teach it. The interviewer said he didn't care. "All you have to do is stay a day ahead of the kids. Besides, you don't have to worry about any of your students going on to college. You don't have to worry about any of them knowing that you don't know. They're just ....junior high kids." I felt he was looking down on those inner city kids. I felt he didn't care about them. He just wanted a body to fill a specific teaching slot.

Since I wouldn't accept that particular position, the man in personnel wouldn't offer me any other teaching job. And there were many openings for which I qualified. I would remember that incident a few years later when I again applied for a job in the Flint Public Schools.

I did accept a job teaching high school English, drama, and coaching debate and forensics in the L'Anse Creuse school district outside of Mt. Clemens, Michigan.

I enjoyed my students. I enjoyed my extra-curricular assignment of coaching the debate and forensics teams. My kids did well. They were super.

But I was naïve. I thought that my drama class should be held in the English classroom that had a stage not in a regular English classroom. The head of the department, a little man in many ways, felt that the room was his. I insisted. The matter went as far as the superintendent, who reluctantly agreed with me. I won the battle but lost the war. I got my classroom with the stage. I also got the ax at the end of the year.

On January 12th, 1960 my wife had an appointment to deliver our first child, but an ice storm hit Mt. Clemens early that morning. So we went slip-sliding down North River Road all the way to St. Joseph Hospital. And with a minimum of fuss, Robert James presented himself to the world. He was a model baby right from the start. Well, almost model. He did teach a young nurse aide the importance of following the simple procedure of placing the fresh diaper over a male baby's wet diaper before removing it. Bob sprayed her as well as the wall. It wasn't polite to laugh. But we did. And she did after wiping her glasses so she could see. We were glad she was just pissed on but not pissed off.

Seven weeks later, Ann was back teaching school. A counselor at L'Anse Creuse High School where I was teaching had died. The current home economics teacher took the counselor's place. Ann was quickly hired to replace her. Later that spring there was the annual Michigan Education Association's conference that MEA members were expected to attend. They closed the schools on that day for that purpose. But I wasn't a member. At that time the MEA was controlled completely by administrators and it was anything but a teacher oriented organization. So I chose not to join. I chose to go to school that day and work. I was there all day working. But that didn't make any difference. The administration docked me a day's pay for not attending the MEA conference. The fact that I spoiled their consecutive streak of 100% membership plaques might have had something to do with it.

Next stop: Mt. Morris High School. Both Ann and I applied for a job there. We were both quickly accepted. Now we had to find a place to live. Since both of us were raised during the big depression, we were very conscious of the costs of buying a house. We decided on what we felt we could afford—something in the neighborhood of $10,000.00. This was 1960. And even back then, $10,000.00 wouldn't buy a new home. The one thing we didn't want to do was to live in a subdivision. We looked and we looked. There were two houses that we seriously considered. One was a house in a racially mixed neighborhood on Avenue B in Flint. It had the advantage of being within walking distance of downtown. The other was an old, old, old dilapidated farm house on 5 acres of land out almost in the middle of nowhere. How old was it? As far as we could determine it was the first house built on that section of land sometime before the Civil War. But it was between two highways. We could walk to a mama-papa grocery store. There was a gas station with a friendly mechanic on the corner. So we opted to live in the country. Since the prices of the two houses were identical and we were very cost conscious, we chose to save a little more money on gas because we were actually one mile closer to the Mt. Morris High School where we would be teaching than we would have been had we bought the house on Avenue B in the center of Flint.

Mt. Morris High School. The building itself symbolized what is wrong with education. It was circular. The classrooms were on the outside. In the center was the gymnasium. Open your class door and you could look down over the balcony seats onto the gym floor.

Ann taught home economics. Along with the college prep English classes I coached debate and forensics as well as being the librarian. It was an interesting combination. Again, I had good students. The poor students, I baby-sat. I might have entertained them, but I sure didn't teach them. I did what was expected of me. I lectured. I made assignments. I corrected papers and handed out grades.

I also became interested in the effect of the power of suggestion in education. One day in my English class, a student asked me if I knew a good way of studying spelling words. I trotted out the old standard method of looking at the word, visualizing the word, writing it down, checking it and writing it again three times.

"But that never works for me," she countered. "I don't have a blackboard in my mind to write on. I can't visualize anything. And copying a word fifteen times doesn't do anything for me either."

So I told her that perhaps she should use the power of suggestion. For demonstration purposes, I had her open a dictionary at random. With her eyes closed she stabbed her finger at a page and hit the word *mendacious*. She had no idea of how to pronounce it or what it meant. So I had her repeat after me the formula that I just made up on the spot.

- I can learn to spell any word.
- I can learn to spell the word *mendacious*.
- It is easy to spell the first syllable: **men**.
- It is easy to spell the second syllable "day" as **da**
- The last syllable is "shus" and that is spelled **cious** just as in pre*cious* and deli*cious*.
- To prove to myself I can learn this word, I will cover up the word and write *mendacious* syllable by syllable.
- I know now how to spell *mendacious* and I always will be able to spell *mendacious*. **Men da cious**.

Then back to the literature lesson we were on. The whole episode had almost completely slipped my mind when three months later, just before the final exams, one of my students asked me if Melinda could still spell that word.

"Of course Melinda can spell the word *mendacious*." That was suggestion #1. "Come on up here Melinda, I know you remember how to spell *mendacious*." That was suggestion #2. "Now show the class that you remember the steps in spelling **men da cious**." That was suggestion #3 and hint, hint, hint by the way I broke it into syllables.

Melinda surprised herself and the class by correctly spelling *mendacious*. But she didn't surprise me. I just knew that there was really something to the power of suggestion. Or the power of teacher expectations. Whichever, whatever.

And then there was Trilby Winn. She was probably the finest student I ever had. She was brilliant. She was a straight A student. She was destined to be her class valedictorian. But she almost self-destructed in my class the last semester of her senior year. One of the English Department's requirements for that class was a book report that would count 25% of the grade. I had told the class that almost any book would be acceptable as long as it was not that kind of book that the parents in this community would object to. If there was any doubt in the matter, they should see me to get approval. Trilby didn't. On the day before the final exam week she handed in her book report on: *The Analysis of Prostitution*. Her first two sentences were: "I have always wanted to be a prostitute. I think that I would make a good one." Talk about getting a reader's attention. Wow! And the rest of the report was better from a purely literary and scholarly perspective. She very adroitly criticized the author for arbitrarily taking the position that members of the oldest profession should receive psychiatric counseling so that they could leave the profession. Trilby stressed the point that the pyschiatric profession should not be passing moral judgments on another profession but rather helping them cope with the stresses *within* their professional and personal life.

What was I to do? I knew that her choice of books to read and report on wasn't going to be accepted unanimously by the Mt. Morris community. But there wasn't time for her to do another book report. Should I give her a zero for a report on an unacceptable book? That was the school's policy. But that would knock her grade from an A down to a C and take the valedictorian honors away from her. Was that right? What to do? I didn't know but I had to make a decision. I called Trilby in and returned her paper in private. I gave her an A. And I told her not to show the paper to anyone. And I told her why.

Well, the next day I was called into the Superintendent's office. Trilby just had to show off her paper to a friend who had to tell her mother who had to tell the superintendent's wife who let him know in no uncertain terms that Mr. McCabe had to be a pervert to give an A to that slut Trilby.

He had a problem. He liked me. He also liked his wife. So, in the course of our little conference, I told him that I was planning to return to school full time that fall to get my masters degree. He sighed a big sigh of relief. Now he didn't have to either defend me to his wife and the board of education nor did he have to fire me.

So my wife, a high school home economics teacher, found another teaching job in the Detroit area so that I could go back full time to the University of Detroit to get my masters degree.

Of all the courses I took, the one that perhaps was the most important was the introduction to research class in which the instructor insisted upon absolute mastery of the essentials. He had a list of over 100 terms and abbreviations commonly used in academic research that had to be mastered in order to pass. In other words, to pass the class you had to demonstrate that you knew such things as *i.e.* meant "that is" and *e.g.* was just an abbreviation for "for example." Today, I find that many people holding Ph.D.'s say "EYE EE" instead of "that is." But I can't look on them as being stupid. They just weren't taught. And after all, I didn't know what *i.e.*, and *e.g.* meant when I graduated from high school *or* from college. I didn't know what these simple common abbreviations meant until I was forced to learn them by a teacher who insisted upon mastery of the essentials. By mastery he meant 100% correct.

And it is that instructor's insistence upon mastery of essentials assumed to be known in graduate school that has affected this dyslexic's way of thinking. Over the years I have slowly come to the simple realization that:

> **Many things need to be taught, not just presented or assumed to be known.**

This class was my first class in which the concept of mastery teaching was employed. Naturally, the instructor was a subject matter expert, and the class was NOT an education class. Not even in the education class that taught the concept of mastery learning was mastery insisted upon.

But perhaps the greatest lesson that this one instructor taught me was not to blindly trust historical facts. He had every member of his class select a different encyclopedia to research the facts about John Milton, the one English poet about which more is known than even William Shakespeare. Each of us had to simply list what happened on every date that was mentioned in the encyclopedia's article about Milton. Then, we made a master chart.

We could hardly believe it. Every encyclopedia reported as indisputable facts dates for certain events in his life, such as birth, death, marriage, and publication of poems and plays that were different from what other encyclopedias reported as indisputable facts. Not one of the books mentioned the possibility that Milton experts were not in agreement. Not one of the articles agreed with any other article for all the dates. There was no way of making sense of it. But it certainly helped us understand that just because something is reported as a fact in an encyclopedia, doesn't make it true.

That instructor's message came back to haunt him. At the beginning of his class on Milton he told the class that God is the hero of *Paradise Lost*. He also admitted that he was a leading authority on Milton and *Paradise Lost* so that no one should even attempt to write a term paper with the thesis that Satan is the real hero.

That was a challenge to me. How do I find a way to convince a Milton expert that he's wrong? Then, in my research I encountered an article written by a nun entitled, "Is Satan an Ass?" That was all I needed. I had both a title that would shock, a reason for using the shocking title, and a hook upon which to base the entire paper. The title? "Is God an Ass?"

The instructor told me afterwards that when he saw my title, he got so angry he almost threw it in the basket without reading it. How could a graduate student in a Catholic university write a paper with that title? But then his curiosity overcame his anger and he read the preface in which I quoted the title of the nun's article and laid down a different framework upon which to judge *Paradise Lost* as a poem and not as theology.

This was in 1958 many years before schema theory was ever advanced in the schools of education. But I already was aware of the fact that our experiences and prior knowledge affect how we look at things and how we interact with written text. So I used as the framework for my term paper a trial using a Buddhist judge, a Shinto prosecutor, a Hindu defense attorney, and a jury composed entirely of non-Christian Japanese. To further eliminate the emotional associations of critical words in the text I substituted "Japanese sounding and looking words" for the Christian words. For example, the *character* "God" in the poem Paradise Lost became Kyo and Satan became Ito. The angels became banyels and the devils became saynids.

At the end of the trial, it was clear to the jury that the *character* Ito displayed those characteristics most commonly associated with heroes and the Kyo very definitely displayed those characteristics most commonly associated with villains.

Instead of throwing my paper into his waste basket, my instructor ended up passing my paper all around the English department at the University of Detroit.

Daring to be different, daring to look at a subject from a different angle seems to be part of my character. So much so that I probably was the first graduate student to deliberately use a taboo word as a one word sentence paragraph in a scholarly paper.

My paper was on the scatology in the writings of Jonathan Swift. My thesis was that Swift used language that was appropriate for his subject matter to forcibly drive home his point. Most critics of Swift took a different position. One critic which I quoted directly in the paper said that "Swift's choice of the word *Brobdingnagian* was prompted by his childhood preoccupation with the drippings and droppings of feces." When I finished that quote I wrote one simple word: "Shit!"

Then I continued on writing in my controlled scholarly fashion. The instructor, who was something of a prude and one who probably never used that word in public, told me that when he read the word *shit*, he broke out into an hysterical laugh of approval. His comment was that he never before encountered a more apt and powerful usage of a common word to make a point.

I finished my masters degree in one year and began looking for a college position. Unfortunately, the positions teaching college at that time paid less than high school teaching positions. We needed some money at that time, so I swallowed my pride and applied once more for a teaching position in the Flint Public Schools.

About the first thing the person who interviewed me asked was had I ever applied to the Flint Schools for a position before. My suspicious mind reacted instantly. I answered, "No." Then the interviewer continued going through my application and apparently was impressed enough with my scholastic record to offer me a teaching position at Flint Northern High School. He handed me the contract which I signed. He signed it. When I got up to go, he shook my hand. Then I dropped the bombshell, "Gee, it was a lot easier this time."

"This time!" he echoed me. "Just a second!" He dashed across the room to a filing cabinet and feverishly flipped through folders. I could read his lips as he said "Damn it."

When he came back he told me my name was in the file of "Never to hire" because I had once turned down a job offer. He just hoped none of his superiors found out that he had goofed and signed me up.

So that fall I started teaching English at Flint Northern High School. The rest of that school year is just a blur in my memory. About all I can remember is that I resented my principal blatantly violating school policy which prohibited prayer in the classroom. But because he was a Michigan Hall of Fame coach, he was allowed to get away with it. He insisted on having someone read over the public address system a passage from the Bible everyday during homeroom period.

Maybe it was some kind of inside joke. Because the P.A. system didn't function. It would sound something like this:

BLATT-TTT Lord is BLATT-TTTTT shall BLATTT-TTT green pastBLATT-tttt.

The P.A. system was never used for anything besides Bible readings that no one could understand. And it was never repaired until after the principal, a sacred cow, retired. And because the P.A. system didn't work, it wasn't used the day John F. Kennedy was assassinated.

How well I remember it. The news that JFK had been shot was given to us by counselors who went room to room saying the bare minimum. I was hoping that my premonition was wrong. I just knew that the press was being lied to or they were lying to us. How could anyone survive a head wound? But I didn't share my dark thoughts with my students. Instead, I tried to reassure them. Then, I continued teaching.

I was reading to my class when the door opened and a counselor poked her head in and whispered those words we didn't want to hear, "He's dead."

I closed my book and just stared. I let my tears flow down my face. I didn't say a word. The class followed my lead. No one spoke. We just sat there in shock. When the bell rang ending class, everyone filed out without saying a word. I just sat there in a trance.

Five days later my wife went to the hospital. And so did my sister Betty June. To the same hospital even. Both on a specialized weight reduction program. Our daughter Linda Carol entered the world kicking and screaming. And not too long afterwards her "twin" cousin Steve put in his appearance. But not before one of the nuns at St. Joseph Hospital was made temporarily speechless. It just so happened that the nun who took Ann up to the labor room while I filled out the paperwork was the same nun who wheeled my sister Betty June up there while her husband Bob was filling out the papers. Ann had just gone into the delivery room and I was on my way to the waiting room when I spotted Betty June.

"Sweetheart!" I exclaimed and rushed up and gave her a big hug and kiss. You should have seen that nun's face. You can imagine what she was thinking. But Betty June just had to put her at ease by saying, "Don't mind him, Sister. He's just my crazy brother."

So the two sisters-in-law shared the same room and were able to show off their "twins" and work together on deciding names. I suggested that Betty name her son Stephen Oliver Szilagyi but she caught the monogram SOS and decided not. Instead she elected to name him after his uncle judge Stephen Roth and grandfather Joseph.

We thought it would be appropriate to name our new daughter after my father who was slowly dying of cancer at the time. None of his seven children had been named after him nor any of his fifteen grandchildren. There was a reason of course. As the youngest boy in his family he had been saddled with the names of the only two uncles that hadn't had someone named after them. One was Uncle Lemuel. The other Uncle Cicero. So he became Lemuel Cicero. A name that rarely appeared anywhere. He was known as Bud or Mac McCabe or just plain L.C. to his friends. My mother never knew his full name until the day she married him. He was just Bud McCabe to her. So when I told dad we had named our daughter after him, he winced.

I said, "No Dad, we didn't name her Lemuel Cicero. That wouldn't be right. So we just gave her your initials L. C. and named her Lucretia Cassandra." And for a minute or two he believed me. He was relieved that we had used plain old traditional names like Robert James for our son and Linda Carol for our daughter. That's what he had done for his seven children.

1. Jack, born in 1926, married Mazie Barone, took over dad's accounting business and provided the financial support for my mother until she died. They had five children: Albert, Mark, Mary Jo, Daniel, and Matthew.

2. Betty, born in 1929, was my mentor. She married Bob Szilagyi. They had six children: Jim, Paul, Teri, JoAnne, Mary Beth, and Steve (Linda's twin).

3. Don (That's me!) born in 1932, married Ann Smith. We had two children: Bob and Linda.

4. Tom, born in 1937, married Wilma Davidson. They had three children: Michael, Patrick, and John.

5. Mary Clair, born in 1941, married Tom Scott. They had one girl, Jennifer.

6. Nan Therese, born in 1946, married Dan Keilitz. They had one son, Kevin.

7. Jim, born in 1952, married Sue Trim. They had two children, Megan and Cameron.

As you can tell from the birth dates that there is a tremendous spread in ages between my brothers and sisters. From the oldest in my family (Jack) to the youngest, Jim, there is 26 years difference. Our mother was 46 when Jim put in his appearance and was a grandmother twice over by that time. When Jim graduated his niece Mary Jo McCabe, who was only a few months younger than he was, stood next to him in line for her diploma too.

The year after John F. Kennedy was assassinated and Linda Carol McCabe and Steve Szilagyi were born, I was transferred to the brand new Northwestern High School. It was beautiful. And the roof leaked even before it opened. It was another example of a building being sold to administrators with no input from the teachers. It had a state-of-the-art air-conditioning system, or so they said. Of course, it only works properly when all the doors to the classrooms are closed. Open doors put a strain on the system. Apparently the architects and engineers who designed it and the administrators who approved it had been out of the classroom for so long they forgot that for five minutes every hour every classroom door is open for the passing of classes.

Chapter 11

Teacher unions: Getting involved.
Getting Punished.

THE LABOR MOVEMENT was slow to arrive in the field of education. When I started teaching there were no effective teacher unions in Michigan. There were teacher organizations affiliated with the Michigan Education Association (MEA) and the National Education Association (NEA) that most teachers belonged to, but they were totally dominated by administrators. So much so, that all teachers were expected but not required to join. When I was at both L'Anse Creuse and Mt. Morris, for example, I elected not to join. Why? Well, that was the exact question I asked my principals. *Why should I join?* Neither principal could list any real substantial benefits for membership other than having one day off for attending meetings. I told them I would rather work than attend boring lectures. Because I was the only one not to join each year, the principals didn't get their 100% membership plaque. And even though I worked that day at both schools, both principals docked me a day's pay.

In 1966 a revolution was taking place within the MEA. The administrators were leaving and forming their own organization. The MEA and NEA began to follow the lead of the American Federation of Teachers (AFT) which was affiliated with the AFL-CIO. When it became apparent to me that the Flint Education Association (FEA) was serious in becoming a union and wanted to represent the teachers in collective bargaining, I joined. The other teacher organization, the Flint Federation of Teachers (FFT) was already vocally militant but small in numbers.

There was a battle for recognition. Guess who belonged to both sides? I was inside both groups and was doing my best to make the leaders understand that it wasn't the other teacher group that was their enemy. It was the administration. Over and over and over I kept hammering away at a very simple concept. No matter which teacher organization wins the right to become recognized as the official representative of the teachers, we should stand united. We should work together. We should not allow the administration to continue to pit each group against the other. Eventually, the leaders on both sides finally began to accept that simple premise. I doubt that they even knew where the idea came from. At any rate, in August, 1969 the FEA joined hands with the FFT and formed a new organization called the United Teachers of Flint. Members had to pay their local dues to the UTF but had the choice of which state and national organization they wanted to join. Flint's UTF became the first and as far as I know the only teacher union that had the two national organizations, the NEA and AFT, united at the local level.

At that time, school administrators tried to break teacher's unions by eliminating their leaders. That is, they eliminated them by promoting them. A former FEA president, Stewart Rowe, the man who talked me into joining the FEA and becoming active in the new teacher organization, was lifted into administration, eventually becoming Personnel Director. Mary Carey, who was president at the time of our first strike, became a principal. Tony Diego who succeeded her, was offered a superintendency in another school district. David Carnegie who followed Diego as president became the principal of my alma mater, Cook School, which by now was no longer the best grade school in town. Me? Well, the administrators did not consider me to be a team player. I had radical ideas. For example, back in 1968 I wrote an article in the union newsletter warning about the dangerous and potentially explosive situation in our large high schools from students in the halls. The article was entitled, "Kiss my ass!" It caught everybody's attention. But it apparently wasn't convincing. Most teachers felt that this language was inappropriate. I agreed. I didn't like having students say to me, "Kiss my ass!" when I stopped them in the hall to ask for a hall pass.

With over 2,000 students, there was no way for me to know them all. And remembering faces from one exposure is impossible for me.

My suggestion was too simple. In my classroom my students behaved. They knew me. They knew I knew them. The students I had in class would behave properly even in the halls. But they composed only 5% of the student body. 95% didn't know me, and they knew I didn't know them. Ergo, they could say whatever they wanted to. They knew a teacher couldn't physically force them to do anything. So "Kiss my ass!" and many phrases far more vulgar and inappropriate were used routinely on teachers who tried to maintain discipline in the halls.

My solution was simple. Basically, the same solution the military has used for years. Name tags. Nowadays factories, hospitals, government offices, retail stores and all kinds of businesses use name tags with pictures. This was much too radical. Student and teacher identification badges! Too radical. Never mind the fact that first year teachers were often humiliated by being told that the teachers' lounge wasn't for students or being reprimanded for not having a hall pass. Never mind the fact that non-students could wander the halls at will. Identification badges for students and school personnel was too radical an idea. McCabe was too radical a union leader. The administration didn't want to get rid of me by making me an administrator. I couldn't be trusted. So, what could they do? They couldn't fire me. I was on tenure. But they could and did begin a campaign to get me to leave of my own accord.

All of a sudden I didn't have all nice twelfth grade college prep English classes. Now I had the lower tracks. Large classes. The worst students. How do you teach kids who can barely read and write?

Again I did a rather radical thing. With the permission and cooperation of the English department I had all the students at Northwestern tested for reading levels and spelling as part of a needs assessment. Then I tabulated everything by track and by race. What I discovered was really predictable. All tracks had a bell curve. There were students in the lower tracks who could read and spell better than most in the upper track. There were students in the upper track that scored well below the average of the lower tracks. My reports were ignored and buried.[1] I believed then and I still believe today that the reason my reports were ignored is that the administration did not want to admit that the educational tracking system they were using ended up as de facto segregation. Or you might say that the school had segregated integrated classes and integrated segregated classes. That is, the college prep classes were 95% white. The non-college prep classes were 65% black. The general classes were 90% black.

Perhaps because I was such a vocal critic of the curriculum in the teachers' lounge and in teachers' meetings, I was asked to serve on the system-wide English textbook selection committee. At the first meeting, the administrator in charge of fine arts, a Mr. Faulkner, gave all the members of the committee three sets of English Literature books for grades ten through twelve for a three track system. Evaluate and choose were his directions. Unfortunately, I spoke up. I told him that he was getting the cart before the horse. We should not let the books we choose determine our curriculum. We should first determine the curriculum and then choose the books we need to fit the curriculum. In the appendix I give a more detailed account of what I had envisioned. One of the things I mentioned was that I had already completed a needs assessment for Northwestern and felt that the results would be much the same at the other high schools. We argued. I was alone in my opinion. But I had a loud voice. I also had a lot of facts. I had done my homework. One by one the members of the committee began to agree with me. Before the meeting concluded we decided not to order any books until a new curriculum had been decided upon, one that would not be an exercise in segregated racial integration or integrated racial segregation.

I wasn't surprised when I was not asked to be on the new English curriculum committee, but I did give them my recommendations.[2] The consultant who ran the committee from his downtown

---

[1]Some of these reports can be found in the Appendix.

[2]These recommendations can be found in the Appendix.

administration office said my talents were needed elsewhere. Sure. You believe that and I have some tokens for the toll bridge connecting San Francisco and Honolulu. He just wanted me out of his hair. Instead of that committee, I was put on the first system-wide remedial reading curriculum committee. Although I had a voice in what was to be taught (the generalities), I wasn't allowed to have a voice in selecting the materials or the equipment necessary for teaching remedial reading at Northwestern High School.

So from teaching the lower tracks I would soon be teaching the lowest track. It would be a challenge. And I had to be certified as a reading teacher by taking 15 credit hours of reading courses.

The only problem was staying awake in those boring classes. In one of the classes, which at least had the practical aspect of involving tutoring a real student, I made the mistake of opening my mouth and saying on the first meeting that, "I can't understand how a student can get all the way to the tenth grade and still not be able to read word one."

I was assigned Michael Wilburn (not his real name). Michael was in the ninth grade. He couldn't read *shit*. Literally. When I first starting working with him, I knew traditional Dick and Jane approaches weren't going to work with him. In his first answer to my first question, Michael said, "I don't give a shit." So I wrote down his answer, "I don't give a shit." All he could read was the word *I*.

Even though I gave him the words *don't* and *give* and *a* Michael still didn't get the word *shit*. This was my first real experience using the highly touted Language Experience Approach (LEA). It also became the start of a technique I would later refine while working in the Flint Regional Detention Center. I would help the illiterates get their *shit* together by starting with the word *shit* making sure they could spell and read the word *shit*.

Starting with the word *shit* is not all that unusual as I later found out by talking to other teachers of the "hopeless." But that technique is not to be found in any courses in teaching remedial reading. Yet, it makes sense. First of all it catches the student's attention and catches him a little off guard. Instead of his normal defensive demeanor he gets sucked into the fun of reading and spelling. And of course I tell my student that I teach backwards. I teach the little word part *it*. I would write it in green ink about ten times. Then I put *sh-* in red ink just in front of *-it* making *shit*. Using color to distinguish the beginning sounds from the ending sound helped. I would ask Michael for a word that rhymed with *shit*. At first he had trouble doing this, but I loosened him up. I would give a rhyming word and ask him what letter he thought started the word. Most of the time he was successful. It was the smile of recognition on his face when he got the word *fit* right that made me realize I was on the right track and that Michael could learn to read through the backdoor of spelling by key words and word families.

I treated the word *shit* as a key word. Any word that starts with the letters *sh* starts just like *shit* whether *shop*, *show*, *shin*, or *ship*. Any small word that rhymed with *shit* would end *-it*.

All the beginning consonants were written in red ink. The ending family sound (in this case *it*) was written in green ink.

shit

it

bit

fit

pit

spit

hit

lit

slit

flit

quit

I also found out that I could successfully use certain types of children's books with Michael. If they were funny. If they could make him laugh, he didn't feel put down. His first book that he ever read by himself was *I Wish I Had Duck Feet.* He was learning that he could learn.

At the end of this summer school session, my instructor asked me to fill out for the school system the traditional form that showed what the student had been taught and with recommendations for further "treatment."

I knew that this form would just be filed. So I approached my instructor and asked him if I could just write in GIANT BLOCK letters.

PLEASE CONTACT ME.

I will work with his teachers and his counselor to plan a very specific course of action. I feel responsible for this young man. I have given him hope. I don't want to see him lose that hope. PLEASE let me help you help him."

Thank you,

Don McCabe   Phone 555-1234

School started. Nothing. Two weeks into the school year I mentioned this fact to the principal of Michael's school who just happened to be on the same committee for solving school problems that I was. He said it would be all right if I initiated the contact. So I did. I called the school and talked to his counselor. I made the mistake of asking to see Michael's records. At this time, I believed what I was taught in my remedial reading courses that school records are a good source of information that can help in tutoring.

Two hours after my call, I was called into my principal's office and roundly chewed out. My principal told me I was interfering with another school's program. His choice of words were colorful. His intention was clear. But I didn't back down. In fact, I played the role of the insulted person to the hilt. All I was doing was my job. Part of my job was to take the reading class. Part of my responsibility in taking the class was follow-up. I was doing my job.

Two hours later, I was called out of class. Now it was the assistant superintendent who accused me of unfair labor practices. As I was a union leader, he suspected me of wanting information on Michael Wilburn to push some secret teacher union agenda.

Here I was trying to help a student continue learning to read. I didn't want him to slide right back into total illiteracy. I explained that over and over to the assistant superintendent. I really believe he eventually believed me. But, *he* was a team player. The administrative team had to be automatically against any teacher union program, real or imagined.

It was at the end of the long confrontation that I pulled my Pontius Pilate act. I told him that I felt responsible for Michael Wilburn. I knew that I could help his teachers help him learn to read. If the school insisted on refusing my help, then the school should take responsibility for whatever happens to Michael Wilburn. I had tried. I washed my hands.

But the blood never really came off my hands. Or to mix another metaphor, Michael Wilburn was to become the albatross which still to this day hangs around my neck. The last time I heard of him was when I read a news article about his release from jail after having spent more time waiting for his trial then the time he would have had to spend if he were to have been found guilty without a trial.

The last semester before my duties as head of the Remedial Reading Department began, Northwestern was really into what they called the Trenton Plan. That was what they called the system of having individual English Courses instead of College Preparatory English I, II, and III, Non-College English I, II, and III, and General English X, Y, and Z.

Although I had originally fought for this plan, it wasn't what I wanted. And I won't take any of the blame for the proliferation of inane courses that maintained the tracking system under the guise of expanded choice.

Had I remained on the committee I would have fought tooth and nail against most of the courses that were put into the English curriculum. But my committee assignment had been changed. I've often been told you shouldn't pray for things because sometimes you get what you pray for. In my case, we did get a completely revamped curriculum that was far worse than the three-tiered monstrosity I had hated. Now we had courses called "Man and the Motor Car" and "Girl Talk" as well as "Ethics" and "Modern Transformational Grammar." The last two were courses that no member of the English Department wanted to teach. So they were given to me.

Ethics was a fun course to teach. Actually, I taught it as a course in logic. My students were expected to be able to identify the major premises for different positions on ethical problems and to understand such concepts as "ends" and "means."

But it was the Modern Transformational Grammar class that was the challenge. How do you teach a subject that no one has either any interest in or use for? I decided to approach the problem head on. My first words to the class were:

You are going to be studying transformational grammar. I'm not going to lie to you. You will never have any use for transformational grammar. The book we will be using is as dull and boring as the subject is itself. But, that's no reason to try to get a transfer out of here.

In the first place, it's too late—and you know that. So I'll tell you what we're going to do. I'm going to teach you how to study.

Almost all of you in this class are going on to college. Believe me, you're going to have some classes with teachers that will bore you to death and books that will put you to sleep if you try to read them. Hopefully, you won't have many. But you are bound to have a few.

What I'm going to do is show you how to study—not as individuals. Boring stuff is almost impossible to learn by yourself. Misery loves company. Company helps alleviate boredom. Company brings challenge. Cooperative studying brings success.

I am going to show you what to do in classes that are boring, how to take notes, but more importantly, how to work in small study groups outside of class. I will only devote fifteen minutes to normal stupid lecture on the subject. The other forty-five minutes I will be floating around from table to table helping you help each other study what was presented just as if you were in a college cafeteria working with your buddies.

The following are just a few of the ridiculous and useless bits of information that my students were expected to learn.

1. There are only two tenses, past and present. (That's right, no future tense!)
2. Sentences are defined as NP + VP + 2-3-1
3. NP's are Det + N.

Need I go on? In any event, when I gave the final examination that was written by the author of the text—not me—, the lowest score in the class was 92%.

I'm sure that had I not had the experience in my high school trigonometry class of sharing all the trig problems with my five friends in study hall and working them out together, I would not have hit upon this particular system of teaching boring and useless material.

Part II, Chapter 12

Teaching the unteachable.

BOB BLOOMER AND I were put in charge of the first remedial reading program at Northwestern. We were given a small room between two classrooms. This room had originally been designed to be an observation room with one-way glass. But regular window glass had been installed. The students from either classroom could look right into and through our room.

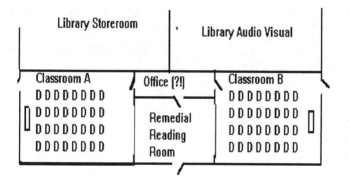

Bob and I were expected to set up a remedial reading program from scratch. However, we had no control over the budget or how the money was to be spent. Downtown administration spent thousands of dollars on books for us to use. They were all designed for grade school kids. Books filled with bunny rabbits and balloons just don't belong in high school. They were demeaning. They were embarrassing. Eventually we were to give away almost all the books given us to grade school teachers at other schools within the system. We convinced the administration that our activities would be distracting the two classes that could see through the glass windows that separated us. Bob and I eventually were reimbursed for most of our out-of-pocket expenses for remodeling the room. We painted the windows and put insulation as a sound barrier and paneled the room to cut down on the sound that filtered in from both adjoining classrooms. We built study carrels. We tested students and began our program.

From the beginning Bob and I agreed not to disagree or to teach one another. He did things his way. I did things my way. He got results. I got results.

One of the ways I got results was by using a word family approach. Just like I used the key word *shit* to teach the *sh* digraph and the *-it* family, I would take whatever word a student was having trouble reading and teach him a whole bunch of words that shared the same pattern. For example, if Albert E. couldn't read the word *advice*, I would have him write the word *ice* in green about ten times. Then I would have him spell different words that rhymed with *ice* and write the beginning letters in red.

ice
dice
nice
lice
slice
rice
price
mice
vice
advice

This technique seemed to really help those extremely poor readers that I worked with. How poor were they? Well, most of them tested out at the beginning between 2.5 and 4.0 reading levels.

Since we had to have reading scores for placement into the program, Bob and I administered reading tests to the entire school. What we found out was not for dissemination.

> 75% of the school's population were technically eligible
> for remedial reading!

At that time any student reading two or more levels below his grade level was considered in need of remediation. The high school's median reading level was 7.2. That meant that well over half the school's student population was technically eligible for remedial reading. The rule was any student who was two or more years behind in reading needed remedial help.

So Bob and I concentrated on those with the greatest need. The vast majority of the students received no special help in reading. They just stumbled through their classes. Many of them dropped out. The others persisted and collected diplomas that they couldn't read.

One day one of my students, Albert Eddy, called me over to his desk where he was doing some silent reading and asked me what a word was. The word was *technique*. I wrote out *-ique*. And suddenly it dawned on me that had the word been spelled *teckneek*, Albert would have been able to read that word. So to test my theory that by this time Albert was pretty good with basic phonics, I wrote out *teckneek*. Albert read it right away.

So I told Albert that he was getting real good at reading words as long as they were spelled the way they should be. I stalled a little bit for time hoping that I could think up a whole bunch of fancy words that ended *-ique*.

I couldn't. My mind just blanked out. At the time, I couldn't think of:

antique
unique
physique
critique
plastique
fantastique
mystique

boutique
Angelique
Monique
Mozambique
pique

The bell rang ending my class. I don't think Albert Eddy realized how embarrassed I felt. All I knew is that I needed a reference book that had word families in it. So after school I walked into the office of the Assistant Principal for Instruction. I explained my problem to Wilton Slocum. I needed a reference tool for word families. Using word families to teach reading and spelling has been used for hundreds of years. I told him that there just had to be a book in which I could look up word families and find all the words that belong to the one I wanted to teach. He agreed. But because it was December, I wouldn't be able to requisition one until the following November and would not be able to receive it until the September following the order period. In other words, I couldn't get it for another two years.

So I told him to forget the requisition route. I would pay for it out of my own pocket and order it immediately. All he had to do was find out the name of the reference tool and the publisher. I would take care of the rest. Sounded reasonable to him. He agreed to locate the reference tool for me. And once a week I bugged him about it. Finally, he told me that there wasn't any point in him looking any more. According to the various educational research centers at the University of Michigan, Michigan State University, Ohio State University, and Columbia University, no such book existed. The reference desk at the New York City Library and the Library of Congress also said the same thing. No such book existed. Damn, damn, damn.

Being a teacher, I had to complain loud and long in the teachers' lounge. And one of my so-called friends just had to bait me with:

"McCabe, you're a linguist. You've got a whole summer off. Why don't you make your own word family book?"

I was just ignorant enough to think I could do it in a summer's time. And I am stubborn enough to have kept at it. It only took me twenty years to complete the project. I now have the resource book I wanted back then. I now have a reference book in which I can look up any word and find all the words that fit the same pattern.[1] For example, I can look up the word *flat* and find on one page all the *-at* words from *cat* to *splat*. Or I can look up the word *fraction* and find all the *-action* words from *traction* to *attraction*. I sure wish that somebody else would have written that book fifty years ago. But nobody had been either as stupid or as stubborn as I was (am?). So I started my simple little task that I thought I could complete in a summer's time. After all, I had managed to put on a twenty by thirty foot addition to our house in a summer's time practically all by myself.

While I was beginning to codify the language by word families, I was beginning to understand more and more about the connection between spelling patterns and reading. But nothing made the strong connection between the two better than the bet I made with the typing teacher Esther Fineberg.

Again, it came about as a result of a teacher complaining in the teachers' lounge. This time it was Esther who was complaining. Normally, teachers complain about their students. Esther wasn't complaining about *them*. She was complaining about *herself*. She felt she was losing her ability to teach. She just couldn't get her students to type with the speed and accuracy she was accustomed to getting.

"Esther," I said, "It's not you. It's your students. You're used to working with students who are good readers. Northwestern is no longer a mostly middle class white school. It's becoming an inner city school. Our students are poor. They're coming out of homes where nobody reads and education is not a high priority. You can't expect to teach them as well as you can teach the others who can read."

---

[1] See pp. 283-285 for explanation of this book, *The Patterns of English Spelling*.

Esther, being a natural believer in racial equality, couldn't and wouldn't make the connection between her students inability to reach the traditional typing standards and their poor reading abilities. She wouldn't buy my theories.

So I bet her a steak dinner that I could predict what grades she gave in typing (give or take one grade level) if all I knew were the grade level reading scores of her students. Esther was hungry for a free steak dinner. She actually went to the students' cumulative records and picked off all the grade-level scores they received in reading in the 10th grade.

When she gave me the list of all her students with the grade level, I just had to try to live up to my big mouth. What I did was to assign the grade of B to all students who were reading at grade level or above. Those students reading one or two levels below grade level I assigned the grade of C. Those students reading more than two levels below grade level I assigned the grade D.

In her five classes I missed on only one student! This was one who could have been an A student but didn't like to come to class more than once a week.

The steak dinner tasted good. But Esther wanted to know *why* the connection. She may not have been a mathematician, but she knew there had to be some causal relationship between reading ability and typing grades. What she wanted to know was why, why, why.

Big mouth McCabe now had to satisfy her curiosity. But how? Well, first things first. I had to put my ideas on paper. Talking about it wouldn't work. In the teacher's lounge you were lucky to be able to string three sentences together before you were interrupted. So I wrote the following:

Good readers have built-in responses to spelling patterns, so they can easily read and spell non-words like: depotion, piction, incordation, and cligging. Good typists are good readers who build quickly upon these built-in responses to develop new patterns.

Good readers already "know subconsciously" the patterns so they don't need training to type by patterns.

Poor readers don't know the patterns and don't know the words so they must type letter-by- letter, stroke-by-stroke.

Poor readers need training in patterns to become good typists.

dGoo rdrseae hvae bltui-ni rspnsseoe ot lpsnlgei pttnsr,ae os htye cna syleai rdea nda pllse nn-o rwsdo lki:e dptneoi,o pctnii,o ncrdtn;kioaio nda cglgngi.i dGoo tpstsyi rae gdoo rdrseae hwo bldui qckylui pnuo htsee bltni-iu rspnsseoe ot dvlpoee wne ptrts.nae

dGoo rdseae lrdyaea knw"o sbcnscsll"yuoiou hte pttrsnae os hyte dnto'ndee trnngaii ot tpye yb pttrsn.ae

rPoo rdrseae dnto'nkwo hte ptrtnsae nda nt'do nwko hte wrdso os hyte mtsu ypte lttree-yb-lttr,ee srtkoe-yb-srtko.e

rPoo rdrseae ndee gtnrnaii ni ptrtnsae ot bcmeoe gdoo tpsyt.si

In the first column, is my theory. The second column contains exactly the same words and the exact same letters with one _small_ change. I deliberately scrambled the letters so that all natural spelling patterns were eliminated.

When Esther typed the first column, she whizzed right through it at about 100 words per minute with no errors. When she tried to type the second column, it quickly became apparent to her that I knew what I was talking about. Her speed slowed down to a virtual crawl (maybe 25 wpm) as she had to think each letter separately and she made quite a few more errors than she thought she did.

Now that Esther knew that I was right in theory, she wanted to know what she could do about it in practice. How could she help her poor readers improve their reading and their typing?

So now I examined the regular typing text from the viewpoint of a poor reader or a student with learning disabilities. On the very first day you were expected to learn nine different key positions, the four home row keys for the left hand and four home row keys for the right hand plus the space bar.

That poses no problem for good readers and people who have no problem memorizing. But how about the poor readers? The LD kids?

And how were the letters presented in the traditional typing text? They were not presented in patterns. For example, when the letter *c* is taught in one such text these are the words used: *c*am *c*old *c*an mu*c*h.

So when I decided to write my own typing text I did two things. First of all I slowed down the presentation. Instead of nine positions on the first lesson. I taught only four. Instead of covering the entire keyboard in only eleven lessons, I used 28 lessons.[1] Secondly, when I presented a letter, I would present it in connection with a specific spelling pattern. This way students would learn not just the position of a key on the keyboard, but a phonic spelling pattern.

---

[1] This typing book is available from the AVKO Foundation. Its title: *Individually Guided Keyboarding.*

Sample Exercise to Demonstrate the Difference

Traditional Text introducing letter h

```
hh hh hj hh hj ha has had had
hh has has a l all all lad he had
huge height ghost spaghetti
```

My Text introducing letter h

hhh sh sh sh ash hash; ash cash;

ash, cash, rash, crash; ash lash flash;

ash rash trash; ash mash smash

I used this concept to write a term paper for a graduate course for a professor who was blatantly anti-linguistic and anti-phonics. I was pleasantly surprised to get a grade of A+ + + + +. Not only did he like my ideas, he wanted me to go with him to Kent State University where he was going to head up their reading program. He wanted me to get my doctorate, and he volunteered to chair my committee. This I might have done. But before I could, he had a heart attack and died.

As the resident "expert" in problems relating to reading, I was frequently asked for help by the more dedicated teachers on staff. And we had a number of fine dedicated teachers. But the strangest request for help came from Betty Calkins who taught the higher level English composition classes. She told me about her student who was extremely bright. He was a straight A student in such subjects as calculus and physics. Her problem was how to grade him because his spelling was absolutely atrocious.

If he had written the last paragraph, it might have looked like this:

Az the rezadint "expurt" in problums realaiting to reading, I was freakwuntly ast for help by the moar dedakayded techurs on staf. An we had a numbur of fien deducaydud teechars. But the srtanjust rekwess for help caim frum Betty Cawkuns who tawt the hier levle English compusishun classis. She tole me abowt her stoodint who was ekstreamly brite. He was a strate A studint in sutch subjiks as calkyoulus and fiziks. Her prablim was how to graid him bekuz his speling was abbsowlootley atrowshus.

He didn't qualify for special help in reading. He was an honor student who could read at the college level. There were no provisions within the school system to give special help to someone who had a severe spelling disability. I agreed to work with him during homeroom. And with just a few minutes everyday working with his writing and showing him the inner logic of our language, the young man learned how to spell. What I taught him then became the basis for the booklet, which I wrote years later, entitled **The Mechanics of English Spelling**.

Basically all I did was to show him that there were two sets of spelling patterns used in the English language. The first set applies to the simple words, the story-telling words of the English language that existed over two thousand years ago when England was populated by savages or barbarians as the Greeks and Romans would call them. They had a simple language with simple one syllable based story-telling words such as: **hunt, fish, farm, tree, birds, bees, deer, sky, dirt, stone, hut, home, run, jump, play, work**, etc. These are the words used in teaching reading in the first three grades along with the single syllable function words such as: *is, was, were, in, out, up, down, by, here, there, who, what, where, when, why, to, from, and so forth.*

The second set of patterns is what I call the "FANCY." These apply to the polysyllabic words that were forced upon the savages who lived in England by a series of conquerors. The first were the

Roman legions. They gave the savages legal terms from the Latin. Then came the Christian missionaries. They imposed religious and medical words from the Greek upon the savages. Then the Norman French came and almost all words related to food (cuisine) were given new names. They imposed their military terminology upon the simple English savages. But most importantly, they imposed the spellings of their words. And these words imposed from other languages such as the French, the Greek, and the Latin contain different spelling patterns. In these words, for example, the "sh" sound that is always spelled -sh- in the story telling words such as fish, ship, shop, and wash is almost never spelled sh in these "FOREIGN" words that have been imposed upon us such as: *"Special missionary chefs are both anxious and impartial."*

It occurred to me that if the young man with A's in calculus and physics had problems spelling because he hadn't been taught these patterns, quite probably a lot of other students had problems with these types of words.

So, with the permission and help of the English Department I created a special twenty sentence dictation spelling test to be given in every English classroom. The idea was to see if there were any specific problems in spelling that needed to be addressed. Each sentence had two or three problem areas or words that had been suggested by teachers. For example, sentence number 14 was made from the words *difficult*, *find*, *often*, *students*, and *studying*. We really didn't know what to expect, but we hoped we would be able to have a better understanding of the nature of the spelling problems our high school students had.

As it turned out, sentence number 14, *"Many students often find studying difficult"* had the greatest and the severest amount of misspellings. Good spellers, of course, had no problem with it. I had expected that maybe 25% of the students would misapply the rule about words ending in *y* and misspell *studying*. It was over 75% who misspelled the word *studying*, usually as *studing*! Every word on the test was misspelled by someone, even the little words like *a*, *I*, *the*, *an*, *and*, *my*, *his*, *her* and *it* were missed by somebody. What stood out was a fact that should have been obvious. 75% of the student body were lousy spellers. 15% per cent were fair. Only 10% could be considered adequate spellers. Since the test did not have any really difficult words, we couldn't tell how many really good spellers we had at the school. My personal estimate would be 5% or less.

What was clear was that 75% of the student body had problems with the "ITZ" and the "TOOZE" and the "THAIR's" adding *-ed's* where they're not clearly heard as in the phrases "*used to*" and "*supposedto*" and misspelling the word "*have*" whenever it was not a transitive verb– usually as "*of*" in "*should have*" or as **hafta** instead of **have to**. And you should **have** known I would **have to have** an example of three different words spelled **h-a-v-e** in one sentence.

How do you correct these misspellings? Some teachers actually had units on specific words or phrases. Most of their kids would pass the test, but eventually they would go right back to their favorite misspellings when it came to writing compositions.

My solution to the problem was a long time coming to me. It took winning another bet of a steak dinner from a teacher of Black History to force me to come to a very simple discovery. What happened was the result of my natural tendency to argue.

This teacher of Black History, Frankie Lawker came storming into the teacher's lounge. He threw 42 test papers on a desk. "I can't believe how stupid my kids are! Can you imagine that 42 black kids actually believe that the white plantation owners had a right to whip their slaves anytime they damn well pleased!"

I tried to calm him down. But it wasn't easy. If you have ever seen a black man with a red face and veins just popping out of his neck, that was him.

He showed me the essay question he had asked his students to answer as part of the test:

> *For what reason or reasons (if any) should the white plantation owners have been able to whip their slaves?*

I began looking at the answers. The following was fairly typical of the answers:

> *Thay shud have wip thay slave for eny reson.*

At first it seemed obvious to me that they meant:

> *They should have whipped their slaves for any reason.*

But then I finally noticed what should have been obvious. Whenever the student meant "should have" they spelled it "should of." Aha! Eureka! I got it, I got it, I got it. I told the teacher, "If they really meant ***should have*** they would have spelled ***have*** as "***of***." What they really meant was **shouldn't** ***have***. These kids are so used to leaving off endings that it didn't occur to them to add the ***n't***. Their visual memories came up with the ***have***. So they just ended up accidentally writing just the opposite of what they meant to say. They really meant to say:

> *They should**n't** have whipped their slaves for any reason.*

He wasn't buying it. No, his kids were just plain dumb and didn't appreciate the evils of slavery.

So I bet him a steak dinner, I could get all those kids to spell ***should have*** when they really meant ***shouldn't have***. He was sure he would win. All I was going to do was dictate two sentences to his two Black History classes. What he didn't count on was the very devious nature of McCabe.

These were the sentences that I chose to give in just plain normal sloppy speech:

(1) You "shooduv" talked to me first.

(2) You "shoodinuh" spit in my face.

Sure enough those 42 kids wrote things like:

(1) You should of talk to me first.

(2) You should have spit in my face.

The very good students had no problem correctly spelling:

(1) You should have talked to me first.

(2) You shouldn't have spit in my face.

The filet mignon tasted great.

It took the winning of the bet over the phrases **should have** (misspelled **should of**) and *shouldn't have* (misspelled *should have*) to combine with my previous experience learning the Russian language through dictation exercises for me to eventually learn a simple truth about spelling:

When you write you are your own secretary. You dictate in your own sloppy speech to the secretary in your computer brain. It is that secretary that needs training.

If schools continue to *only* teach by word lists that students study, we will continue to have a large percentage of students who misspell common ordinary phrases. The following is a sampling of the types of phrases that need to be taught via the student self-corrected but teacher dictation method:

Sounds like:	Should spell	common misspelling
WUR	we're (we are)	were
THAY'r	they're (they are)	there, their, thair
THAY'r	their	they're there thair
THAY'r	there	their they're thair
YOR GUN nuh	you're going to	your gonna
WUD uh yuh	What do you	What you
WUD juh	What did you	What you

Suh POH stuh	supposed to	sposta or suppose to
YOO stuh	used to	usta or use to
SHuuD uv	should have	should of
SHuuD in uv	shouldn't have	should have
IT soh HAH't	It's so hot	It so hot
IT STOO bad	It's too bad	Its to bad
WAH nuh	want to	wanna
foh'r GRAN it	for granted	for granite
THAT SOH Kay	That's okay.	That okay

It was about this time that I first heard about the concept of "invented" spelling. At first it sounded extremely reasonable. And it is. I do allow it in my teaching and my tutoring, but not just as an end in itself. More about that later. See Chapter 24.

What made me alter my position on "invented" spelling was a happening. Mrs. Betty Josephson, a minister's wife, walked into my homeroom one day with tears in her eyes. But they weren't normal tears. That I could tell by the way she was biting her lip to keep from laughing out loud. She walked up to me and handed me a note with this simple explanation.

"I just couldn't stay in my room after reading this note. It's not polite to laugh in a student's face. Can you translate this?" And she handed me the note.

> Dere techr,
> Ples ekcuss my Johnny.
> He had go doktur get his
> angel raped.
>   His mother

After I stopped laughing, I translated: "Dear teacher, please excuse my Johnny. He had to go to the doctor to get his ankle wrapped."

I know I shouldn't have laughed. But Betty Josephson and I at least didn't laugh in front of her student. It wasn't quite the same as when I was in the 5th grade and the entire class laughed about my "invented" spelling of **_shirt_** in which I somehow managed to leave out the letter **_r_**.

Part II, Chapter 13

My principals and their principles.

THERE'S NO GOOD REASON to list all the principals I served under and to mention my opinion of the principles they used to run their schools. I'm not much for libel suits. So, almost all the names I use in this book are fictionalized. The events may or may not have happened at the school that I mention. But these events, however fictionalized, had a profound effect upon my outlook and my attitude toward the need for educational change.

My first principal at Northwestern, Dr. Motley was smooth. He knew how to handle irate parents. During the first week that Northwestern opened, a mother stormed into his office complaining about that illiterate slob Mrs. Jones teaching her daughter's home economics class. She even had the audacity to give Dr. Motley two days to take care of the situation before she called the school board member, Leo Soda, who was her brother-in-law. Dr. Motley quietly assured her that if what her daughter said was true, she would be gone the next day. Not to worry. These things happen.

So what did Dr. Motley do? He transferred Mrs. Jones from the home economics class and had her teaching the lowest track of remedial English! Those students wouldn't know that she couldn't read and certainly wouldn't complain. Like most school administrators then and now, the rights of those students who need the most help are the last to be considered. It was more expedient to quickly satisfy the immediate whim of a parent with clout than to ensure that students with severe reading problems received the help of a specialist. Instead, they got the illiterate Mrs. Jones. Then, to get a home economics teacher he had the personnel department transfer the remedial reading teacher to Zimmerman Junior High to teach home economics there and to bring the experienced Zimmerman home economics teacher to Northwestern. That's how my wife came to be teaching at Northwestern. And Mrs. Jones? Well, after putting her where she couldn't cause him any trouble by teaching remedial English to kids who didn't care, Dr. Motley carefully documented her illiteracy. He took a fair number of candid photographs showing her slip showing, her room a mess, and even a library card on which she misspelled her own name. Since this was her first year in the Flint system, Mrs. Jones was pink slipped. So she applied to the neighboring Beecher School District for a job. She was accepted after Dr. Motley gave her a recommendation. I never found out what happened to Mrs. Jones. But it is a sad commentary that a person can become certified as a teacher and not be able to read and write. And that has been happening in our colleges of education under the guise of affirmative action.

My second principal was a nice enough man, Mr. Toddy. His biggest problem was that he had as his immediate boss Dr. Motley, the first principal at Northwestern. Any change of any school policy by Mr. Toddy could be construed by Dr. Motley as criticism of how he ran the school when he was principal.

Keeping that in mind, perhaps you can understand why Northwestern was trashed by a large portion of its student body in the following incident.

Just as I can vividly remember where I was and what happened around me the day John F. Kennedy was assassinated, so too I can remember only too vividly what happened after Martin Luther King, Jr. was murdered. The morning after King's assassination, my wife and I got up much earlier than usual. We both had a feeling that the black students might riot.

As we drove past one of Clio's elementary schools, we noticed that the flag was flying high. As that school had no blacks attending it, we knew there wouldn't be any trouble at that school. As I told my wife, if the flag wasn't at half-mast at Northwestern there would be hell to pay. So I stepped on it.

When I pulled in the driveway, I couldn't believe my eyes. No flag was flying at all! Jesus Christ! I whipped my car into the nearest slot, ran to the door and flew down the halls to the main office. I walked by (almost over) the school secretary who guards the narrow passageway that separates the lobby where the teachers' mailboxes are and the office area which teachers entered only with permission.

"You can't go in there!" she screamed after me as I walked straight into the principal's office. Without saying "Good morning," or "Excuse me" or waiting for any of the administrators to speak to me, I just blurted out:

"Get the goddamn flag up at half mast now or all hell is going to break loose!"

"Calm down, Mr. McCabe," Mr. Toddy said quietly. "We know what the situation is. We're in communication with Dr. Motley and his staff downtown. They're having a meeting right now discussing what we should do."

"Fuck downtown!" I screamed at him. "If you don't do something now and I mean NOW not five minutes from now, you won't have diddlely shit left here!"

"You said your piece. We heard you. But we have to do everything by the book. Good bye, Mr. McCabe and thank you for your concern." With that (and two assistants that outweighed me by about fifty pounds), Mr. Toddy firmly dismissed me.

On the way back to my room I passed through the teachers' lounge and warned the teachers there that the administration was sitting around waiting for a decision from downtown as to whether or not to fly the flag at half-mast. I told them that they had better stay close to their rooms and be prepared to lock their doors.

The few teachers who did listen to me were glad they did. Because within ten minutes all hell did break loose. The scenes in L.A. that were captured on video tape of the riot after the police were found innocent of beating Rodney were about the same. Blood and destruction were everywhere.

Whether or not it could have been avoided, we'll never know. But I was pissed then, and I'm pissed now just remembering it. Sitting around discussing whether or not to show respect to a slain civil rights leader instead of just going ahead and doing the decent thing is typical of bureaucracies.

Our next principal was Dr. Wish. He had authored a book on violence in schools. He was an expert. He would solve the problems at Northwestern. He lasted two years.

It was during his administration that a fight broke out in my classroom between two girls. The room had been very quiet as the class was taking a written test. But one girl, Martha K. had been fiddling with Debra J's hair. Debra J. suddenly stood up spilling her desk and books and began assaulting Martha. The noise and the screams brought Tony Diego bursting through the door that connected our rooms. Tony took one. I took the other. Tony took Martha down to the dean's office while I held Debra and tried to calm her down.

Dr. Wish eventually came onto the scene and in all his wisdom asked in front of the girl what I wanted as punishment. I hadn't expected to be put on the spot. But I improvised. "Number one, I don't want an apology from Debra or Martha. I hate phoney apologies. Two, I expect that they be suspended immediately. Three, I don't expect that they be allowed to return until they have written an acceptable apology to themselves and to their parents."

Dr. Wish was aghast. Debra was confused. "What do you mean write an apology to myself?

I told her to think about it. Think about what might have happened. What might have happened to you as a result of the fight. Just think about it. Then write a letter to yourself. And don't forget about your parents. They raised you, didn't they? Think about what could have happened and then write your letter.

They both did. But it took them almost a week. And by the way, I found out that this wasn't the first time for these good friends to get in a real heavy fight. The summer before Martha had stabbed Debra and came fairly close to killing her! Years later Debra became one of the first black female police officers.

Then came our first token black principal, Sidney P. Collins. He was something else. It seemed to me that the administration deliberately set out to find the *biggest* and the *dumbest* black man they could find. They selected an ex-Chicago Bear lineman who somehow managed to have a college bachelor's degree and teacher certification given to him. Most of the black teachers were happy with him, *at first*. The few black teachers that I confided in didn't want to believe me that he was picked because the administration wanted to demonstrate that a black principal wouldn't be the answer to Northwestern's problems.

How bad was he? Well, he lived up to just every negative black stereotype possible. You name the stereotype, and I can recall an incident illustrating it. Our supreme court justice Clarence Thomas had far fewer accusations of sexual harassment and incompetence than Sidney P. Collins. Eventually Sidney did receive a lateral transfer to a position where he had very few papers to shuffle, fewer contacts with female personnel, and no contacts with female students. But before he was transferred, he was brought to my remedial English classroom by the Dean of Instruction who wanted him to know about the new techniques and materials I was developing.

Fat Albert (This is what the students referred to him as) listened politely as I showed him how I helped my students learn to read and spell via word families. Then he asked me a question I'll never forget.

"That's all well and good, Mr. McCabe, but what do you do to help them with their grammar? When they get to college they have to know enough to write 'why come' instead of 'how come.'

Here I am working with high school students reading at the third and fourth grade levels, and my principal, Fat Albert, is concerned about readying them for college! I could just see Fat Albert when he was in college on his football scholarship. He probably wrote something for his freshman composition teacher in which he asked a question using the format, "If that is common knowledge, then *how come* I don't know it?" His English instructor probably slashed at the phrase "*how come*" but hit mostly the *how*. Then above the slashed out phrase he wrote the word *why*. Fat Albert probably misinterpreted the correction. Now instead of writing simply the word *why* instead of *how come*, he writes *why come*.

His spoken language was almost ghetto perfect. He was a Weebee. "We be a fixin' to learn our students how to git ahead."

It was during Fat Albert's short reign that a group of black students came to me for advice on how to form a black student organization. And that occurred shortly after a group of black students had vandalized the Dewater's Art Center at Flint Junior College. They had called themselves the Black Student Union. So I told my students that their chances of becoming a recognized legitimate student organization with the name Black Student Union were about a thousand to one against. But, if they played their cards right, they could slip one by the administration. All they had to do was to form a club with a temporary membership and temporary constitution. Once the club became a reality, then the club members could choose a name more reflective of the club's purpose.

On my desk happened to be a copy of the African writer Fanon's *White Masks on Black Faces*. In the name Fanon I recognized the possibility of an acronym: *F*or *A*ll *N*egroes *o*f *N*orthwestern. I explained to them that Fanon was a famous black writer fighting for civil rights in Africa. Hence the acronym. They liked it. And away they went trying to form the club. And they did. For the first meeting I was their faculty advisor. That didn't last long though. Another teacher, who up to that point had been a good friend of mine, expressed his opinion to the students and the other blacks on the faculty, that I had no right helping the black students. Only a black teacher should help them. And to give a name like Fanon for a black student organization was highly inappropriate. He thought Fanon was a white South African! When I told him that Fanon was a black civil rights activist, he told me, "I knew that." Now he maintained that Fanon was inappropriate because he was an African Black instead of an African American. Oh, well.

But before I and all other non-blacks were shut out, I did give them a list of options for ways of promoting racial equality. Among the options was calling attention to the need for entry-level jobs in the retail businesses in Flint by having shop-ins at stores that had no black employees. I still feel this would have been even more effective than the lunch counter sit-ins. This might have even gotten national media attention. Can you imagine a store catering to almost exclusively rich white women being filled with Black student "shoppers" discussing which 25¢ item they should buy? Can you imagine all these Black shoppers eventually finding very, very inexpensive items and lining up in front of the cashier. This would have ended up in a boycott by whites. This technique was completely lawful. But it was never used. The new faculty advisor for the club preferred discussions and social activities over political action. The club eventually fizzled out after the bulk of the members tired of hearing his bitter anti-white rhetoric and that of the others who tried to out anti-white their sponsor. They also were aware that he had assaulted me in the teachers' lounge not once but twice. The administration refused to do anything to discipline him. I complained to my union because he was my union representative. They refused to do anything. I was told that if I had attacked Fred, I would have lost my job. But since Fred was black and I was white, well that was different. No. It wasn't. It was still a racist position. Underneath the liberal veneer was the belief that Blacks can't be held accountable for their actions in the same manner as whites. To me, that is contemptible condescension. Up to that point, I prided myself on only hating the evil things people do and not the people themselves. Now I discovered I could hate a person even if he were Black.

After I had completed my first editions of *Word Families*, *Sequential Spelling*, and *Reading via Typing*, I tried to get them field tested by other teachers by going through channels. Ring-around-the-Rosie. Promises, promises, promises. Delays upon delays. Supposedly everything was finally approved by the legal department and paper was budgeted for making copies for the junior and senior high remedial reading teachers. Then I got sick and was out for four months. The best the doctors could do was to use the big Latin word lymphocytosis for my condition. And that is simply too many white blood cells. My body was busily manufacturing them to fight off something. But the doctors couldn't determine what it was. All I knew is that I had no energy. Sometime during the summer my strength began to come back.

When I was able to return to work in September, everything related to the remedial reading project had been canceled. I was transferred to a junior high to teach regular low level English classes. This I did, but I still used the opportunity to test the students for spelling problems and for methods of teaching spelling. The sequential spelling and dictated sentences worked very well with these students. Even the top students enjoyed the challenges.

Apparently the administration decided that it was time to really punish me. The next year I was re-assigned. This time I was sent to the hell-hole of the Flint Public Schools which was euphemistically called the Alternative Junior High. These students had no alternative. You see, at that time the administration had the mistaken notion that if each junior high principal had the right to pick ten students they never wanted to see again, their schools would run smoother.

The man who ran the school, Kurt Soper, wasn't given the title of principal. He wasn't qualified—on paper that is. He was qualified to sail any ship on the ocean, but not command a little school. Uh, huh.

As it turned out Kurt was the only principal whose judgment in things educational that I ever respected. He ran a ship which was both tight and loose. Tight where it needed to be. Loose where it had to be to be effective. You would think as principal of such a small and specialized school, he would be able to pick and choose his staff.

Uh, uh. No way. He had to take whoever was given him. He received the refuse of the school system, both students and teachers. Thank God, he had a small core of student counselors that were damn good at their jobs.

It was while I was at the Alternative Junior High that I honed my teaching skills. It was here that my materials and techniques faced the acid test of the hundred most unwanted junior high students in the city of Flint. When I tested them in the fall the median reading score was 3.5. Only two students were reading at grade level.

Although we had very few girls, as would be expected, we did have the only truly integrated school in the city of Flint. When you scrape the bottom of the barrel, race is not really a factor. Gender is.

The materials I had to work with were odds and ends. There wasn't a specific curriculum for English. I was allowed to do my thing. And that I did.

I had a folder for each student with his name on it. As they came into the room, they had to pick up their individual folder and take it to their assigned seat. The moment the bell rang, I began the Sequential Spelling. Then I had two sentences for dictation. The students had to correct their own papers, immediately. They received A's if they made all the corrections. They got an E if they missed correcting one. It didn't take long for them to become accurate at correcting their own mistakes.

Above the chalkboard I had printed a sign that read:

Adult language is not See Spot Run
Let's learn to read and spell adult words.

Everyday I put on the bulletin board a new word strip. One day it might be *filet mignon*. Another day it might be *chateau*. Another day it might be *solder* or *lingerie* or *salve* or *chef* or *solenoid*. To help motivate the students into learning "big" words, I offered $1.00 to the first student to find one of the words in regular printed materials such as a newspaper, magazine, or catalog. Reference materials such as dictionaries, encyclopedias, atlases, etc. would not count.

When a student brought in a word, he got his dollar and his name was printed on the word card. One student in particular really tried to supplement his income by finding words. He ended up going from a 4th grade reading level to the 11th grade level in the course of the school year. He got really turned on to words. And that's what it really takes.

From the moment the word list hit twenty-five words, I offered another monetary motivation for learning. If a student could correctly read fifteen of these adult words in a row he received a quarter. If he could read all of them, he received a dollar. Ten minutes before each class hour ended, the students would quickly put away their individual work and their folders. That's when they had the opportunity to earn money. Almost all the students paid close attention as the better students tried to read fifteen in a row. They were self-correcting their own guesses internally while following along as a student tried to earn his money. I averaged giving out about five dollars a week to the students. This was cheap. But the Flint school system just couldn't adopt that. In fact, it's doubtful that any school system, no matter how rich, would adopt such a simple method of teaching vocabulary. They would rather spend thousands of dollars on deadly boring vocabulary books than spend a few hundred dollars in award money to students.

I did have a number of rules that were slowly introduced to my classes. It was these rules that later enabled me many years later to formulate the "Patterns of Speech" that was made into a book which I entitled: *Get out of my face! Get off of my case!* It is a how-to book for those teachers, counselors, administrators who would like to find a way to help students acquire new patterns of speech that will enable them to avoid violent confrontations as well as helping them develop self-esteem.

It basically started with the first, "Hey man, you gotta..." to which my initial reaction was, "No *boy*, I don't gotta.." Confrontation time! The counselor on hand to help me with my twenty-five darlings was ready to step in and protect me.

But I defused the situation with a very simple, "If you really want me to do that for you, all you have to do is to not start off calling me, "Man." That pisses me off. You don't like being called, "boy." That pisses you off. I won't call you *boy* if you don't call me *man*. Agreed? Secondly, don't tell me what I have to do. That's bossing the boss. I don't like to take orders any more than you do. You don't have to beg. Just ask politely and who knows, I might just do what you want me to do for you. But if you tell me I gotta do it, you can bet your bottom dollar I won't."

So on the spot I turned the young man's demand into a practical psychology lesson on how to get someone to do something for you. What I told him is that getting what you want in life is much like scoring runs playing baseball. You don't want to strike out. And you can't get on base if you have three strikes against you. The moment you say, "Hey!" it's "Strike one!" If you use the wrong name, whether it's *boy, man, you, girl, Mac, buster,* or whatever, it's "Strike two!" And if you order or demand what you want, it's strike three.

Most of the class could see where I was coming from. The grabbing somebody's attention with "Hey," and using a name the other person doesn't like is starting with two strikes against you. Demanding instead of asking doesn't work. Asking instead of demanding might work, but not half so well as if you didn't already have two strikes against you.

How to avoid those first two strikes? Simple. To avoid the first strike, address the person the way he wants to be addressed. If he wants to be called Mr. Smith, call him Mr. Smith. Don't call him Tom. Over and over I hammered the point that if something is worth asking for, it's worth asking for it right.

Then give a reason. Tell the person why you need what it is. Get the person in the mood to help you out. People do like to help others. But people don't like to be told what to do. If they want to help you first, then when you ask for a specific thing, they're much more likely to oblige. For example, "Excuse me, Mr. Jones. My grandmother just went in the hospital, and we don't know how long she's going to live. I would really appreciate it if you would let me leave a few minutes early. I'll make it up tomorrow. Okay?"

Because most of my students had strong behavioral problems, it was very difficult for them to follow the pattern of (1) correct address, (2) reason, (3) request. Their habits of blurting out an order without or before giving the reason were very difficult to break. They needed practice, practice, and more practice.

The concept was easy enough for them to understand. Good salesmen and good con men always make you want to buy *before* they tell you the cost. What my students needed to be able to do is get their boss (or teacher) to want to help them *before* they know what the cost is. Giving a reason after the request is often too late. A boss (or teacher) rarely changes his mind. A good boss often makes up his mind in a hurry. If he hears the request before the reason, he might decide not to grant the request. At that point, before the reason is given, it's all over.

When a student violated a rule that would normally mean staying after school, I did allow them to talk me out of it if they followed the secret formula of (1) correct address, (2) reason, and (3) request. If the student slipped up and got one of the steps wrong or out of order, he could go back to his seat, sit for ten seconds, and then try again. Sometimes it would take six or seven tries before he would get it right.

Part II, Chapter 14

Breaking away, Forming the AVKO Foundation, and BINGO!

IN 1973 I KNEW I had to make a decision soon about the materials I was in the process of developing and testing in the classroom. I knew the materials and techniques worked. I also knew that the administration of the Flint Public Schools did not want to help me. They were not at all interested in solving a reading/spelling problem. To do so they would first have to admit that one existed. This they were not about to do.

As I mentioned in Chapter 11, the downtown school administration and the school board so hated dealing with The United Teachers of Flint (the teacher's union), that they tried to kill it with "kindness" to its leaders. That is, they kept finding administrative paper shuffling jobs for the top leaders of the union. Promotion to administration meant they were now out of the union and onto their side. Stewart Roe was the first effective union leader. He was the first to go. He eventually became the Personnel Director and the highest paid administrator next to the Superintendent. The next union president, Mary Carey, who was the titular head of the union when we had our first strike, was taken out of the teaching ranks and made a principal. Tony Diego, who was the real strike leader and the third president somehow was given an offer he really couldn't refuse, an assistant superintendency in another school district a hundred miles away. The fourth president, David Carnegie, became the principal at my alma mater, Cook School. And the union board member who leaked all union plans to the administration became the Curriculum Director.

At the time I didn't want to believe that the administration and the board of education would stoop to such tactics. I was somewhat of an innocent Don Quixote. Dyslexics tend to be that way. I had seen to it that in our first contract there would be a planning committee composed of administrators and teachers. I was on it. The teachers tried to get the administrators to work with us. They didn't. Nothing ever was done except to have meetings. Their attitude was everything must come from the top down. Teachers weren't about to tell them what to do. We did, but they didn't.

From the time I was stripped of my 12th grade college prep classes and given only the worst classes to teach until I left the school system, I applied to go to the Michigan Reading Association conferences. The only time I went I had to take personal leave and pay all my own expenses. While there I saw who attended. All those administrators who had anything to do with the downtown reading department and who wanted to party went.

I was told that they went instead of teachers because they were in the position to share with teachers the things that they learned. Sure. The only thing they ever shared with me was a simple screening test that gave an approximate reading level. And I was already aware of that one.

I received a lot of promises. It didn't matter what I did or how well I did it, there was always this invisible stone wall. I just knew I could help kids learn to read. I knew we could set up a good working remedial reading program. But downtown had other ideas. But not one of those ideas was to promote me like they had the other key union leaders.

During my last year at Northwestern I had decided that the best way for me to go was to create a non-profit tax-exempt organization to be the vehicle for my research. And so I did with the help of David O'Connell (whose two children I helped overcome their reading problems), Tom Schott, who helped us (and himself) by running a bingo to help raise money for our development needs, Elmer Whaley whose hyperactive dyslexic son with an attention disorder deficit I tried to help, and Alberta Smith, a concerned parent. Later on, at a district level reading association meeting, I met Devorah Wolf quite accidentally. She was listening to me try to explain some of my concepts to a speaker after a session. When she saw my first prototype of my word family book, her eyes just lit up. And I think they have stayed that way through the years. She became a member of the AVKO Foundation's board of Directors and has served over ten years as its president.

Just as a chance encounter led to Devorah's joining AVKO, so too did my first meeting with Mike Lane. But that wasn't at a reading association meeting. No. It came as a result of my disturbing the peace—Mike's peace. He and his young family had moved into the house next door to us. He was up on the roof of his garage laying shingles. As he tells it, when he could hear my voice caterwauling as I was pounding on my piano, he knew that anybody who sang so loudly and so badly had to be Irish and had to appreciate the taste of the good stuff. So he climbed down off the roof, grabbed two six packs of beer from his refrigerator, and walked up and pounded on my door. When I came to the door, I saw a giant of a man with long red hair and a bushy red beard standing with a six pack in each hand who just simply greeted me with, "Hi. I'm Mike your next door neighbor. I just figured anybody who can sing as loud and play a piano as badly as you do needs a beer."

He was right. And I guess my dog Cleo needed a friend, too. His dog Baron, a border collie, came along with him and immediately made friends with my German Shepard. They were such good friends that on cold winter nights, our Cleo would go get Baron, who usually slept in their sheltered breezeway, and bring him into our house for a sleep-over. And protect our property! Whew, no one dared take anything. His wife Karen found out how protective our two dogs were when her parents came one afternoon to pick up her two kids, Molly and Danny. They had no problem going into the house. They wouldn't have had any problem leaving the house, except they each were taking a child. Cleo said, "NO YOU DON'T!" with her unmistakable growl and baring of her teeth. Baron followed suit. Karen had to come out and let the dogs know everything was okay.

Later on both Molly and Danny had occasion to receive help from AVKO. Both the Lane children were (and are) extremely intelligent. But Molly had a rather severe case of dysgraphia by the time she reached the eighth grade. Her spelling was atrocious. Her score on the spelling part of the standardized tests given in that grade put her in the bottom one percentile. Her teachers just couldn't believe that a girl who could read at the college level, had an I.Q. over 130, and scored in the 99th percentile on every other part of the standardized tests could be such an atrocious speller.

That summer she and her younger brother Donald received free tutoring from AVKO. She most likely will graduate valedictorian of her class. For Donald, who had been diagnosed as learning disabled and ADHD (Attention Deficit and Hyperactive Disorders), it's still a bit too early to predict. But it would not surprise me if Donald graduates with honors when the time comes. His reading and spelling abilities have been rapidly increasing ever since he took advantage of AVKO's free tutoring.

So, with the help of my wife Ann, Dave O'Connell, Tom Schott, Alberta Smith, Dan Dolan, Aaron Miller and Elmer Whaley, the AVKO Educational Research Foundation was born. When we came to decide upon a name for our non-profit organization, we wanted the name to really reflect what we were attempting to do and the fact that it was non-profit. The words Educational Research and Foundation came quickly to mind. But it still needed something in front. We said no to both the National Educational Research Foundation and the American Educational Research Foundation on the grounds that they were far too pretentious. And we weren't about to name it after one of us making it something like the Schott Educational Research Foundation or the McCabe-Dolan-O'Connell Educational Research Foundation. Then it occurred to me that since the most of the techniques and materials we were developing incorporated multisensory techniques, we could call it the VAKT Educational Research Foundation after the Visual Audio Kinesthetic Tactile multisensory approach.

I never did like the term VAKT. To me, it's harsh sounding. Besides, I never believed there was enough difference between the terms kinesthetic and tactile to make the distinction. Besides, we often learn as we are talking. So why not substitute Oral for Tactile. But that spells VAKO which might be sounded too much like Wacko! Then my dyslexic mind happened to reverse the letters VA and then we had AVKO. We liked it. For a change we all quickly agreed. And so the AVKO Educational Research Foundation would become our name.

We incorporated as a non-profit organization and received our tax-exempt status. The Bingo that Tom Schott started helped some, but it soon became a drain on my energy. Teaching school, doing research and writing, and running a Bingo was too much. Something had to give. Since our union contract had the provision for an unpaid educational leave of absence for its teachers, I thought there would be no problem getting one to work one year full time for the AVKO Foundation. I checked with the union. I was entitled by the contract. I checked with the administration. No teacher had ever applied for it. So I applied for it. All summer I waited for an answer. No answer. So I called. I was told I couldn't have it unless I showed them that I was enrolled in a doctoral program! That wasn't in the contract. The contract stipulated that I could have a year off for either school or for doing educational research. I was ordered to report to school. I told them I was entitled to the sabbatical by contract, and that I had already committed to the educational research. So I went to my union. What a joke! They wouldn't back me unless I went back to teaching and went through the formal grievance process while teaching!

So I quit.

But did that stop the Flint School system from trying to get to me? Not by a long shot.

They tried to get back at me through my wife. The following is unbelievable but true. On the second Tuesday in September after I quit, my wife Ann was called out of her class and told to see the principal. He told her that she was to report to Longfellow Junior High first thing in the morning. She had four hours to pack up all her teaching materials that she had accumulated in the thirteen years of being the head of the Home Economics Department since

Northwestern had opened its doors. She tried to get the union to intervene.

Do as you're told and then file a grievance was the union's response. Hmm. So she reported. Her new position had five different subject preparations including, would you believe, Boys' Physical Education. Her tears helped only a little. They took away Boys' Physical Education and gave her another different subject to teach.

Before her grievance was heard, she was transferred again to another school. She filed another grievance and before that was heard, she was transferred to yet another school. Strange! And the union didn't help her at all. Stranger yet. Our daughter Linda who was in the ninth grade at the time even wrote a letter to the union on her behalf. It was a strong, hard-to-stomach lesson for Linda, the idealist. How could this happen in Flint, home of the first sit-down-strike, home basically of the union movement?

That was when I realized the truth in the little poster a close friend of mine had given to me.

> # Just because you're paranoid
> # doesn't mean that
> # they're not out to get you!

Getting AVKO rolling wasn't easy. My son Robert was a real help. He could have been one of the last to be hired by General Motors, but instead he chose to help his father and went to work for AVKO. To purchase the needed office equipment and to pay him what amounted to just about half what he would have received from GM, I had to withdraw all the money I had paid into my state retirement fund. And that wasn't enough. So AVKO borrowed money from the bank and I had to put my house (which I owned free and clear at the time) up as collateral. The interest rate was 11%. That AVKO could handle. Then, the interest rates shot up. Before we knew it and before we could reduce the principal on the $18,000.00 loan, the rates climbed all the way to 24%.

Oh well, the Federal Reserve stopped inflation. Yep. Sure. And they also caused a large number of small businesses to go into bankruptcy. AVKO didn't go bankrupt. But AVKO couldn't grow and the McCabe family bank account and savings accounts quickly dwindled.

But, as I have said to my friends and supporters many a time over the years, I am a developer of materials, a developer of techniques to teach reading and spelling, and I am a teacher. A businessman I am not.

Through the first few years AVKO had a few underpaid employees. But there was the problem of increasing sales. To do so we would have to advertise. The board thought we should use a professional. So a professional we hired. The result was the most expensive brochure and mailing we have ever had. It was also the least productive. Back behind the financial eight-ball. Eventually the small grossly underpaid and overworked staff left. And we had to make do entirely with volunteers.

But before that time came, we tried to promote our concepts by exhibiting at various educational conferences and trying to get such organizations as the International Reading Association, The Reading Reform Foundation, The Orton Dyslexia Society, and the Learning Disabilities Association of America to let me speak at their conferences. Well, it's been 21 years since we started. I was able to

134

speak once at the IRA national and once at one of their regional conferences, twice at the Reading Foundation's national conference but never at any local, state, or national conferences of either the Orton Dyslexia Society or the Learning Disabilities Association of America.

It isn't because we haven't tried. We have. These organizations are always quick to ask us to spend money advertising and exhibiting, but slow to accept the fact that we are not a commercial publishing house but an educational research oriented membership organization trying to disseminate its findings, its techniques, and yes, its materials.

One year my son and I drove to Cincinnati, Miami, New Orleans, Minneapolis, Boise, San Antonio, and San Francisco to exhibit at one or the other of the big national association meetings. By far the most interesting trip was the one to San Francisco. My son Bob never needed to become a Boy Scout. He always is prepared. For that trip he even had a tow rope just in case we got stranded in the middle of nowhere and couldn't call a tow truck. He had extra pints of oil, matches, markers, flares. You name it, he had it packed somewhere.

Since we packed all kinds of sandwiches, fruit, and soda pop, we didn't waste any time stopping for meals along the way. We were making such good time that we would have the time to stop and play tourist somewhere along the way. Bob said he wanted to see the giant Sequoia trees. Ever since he read about George Sequoia, the Cherokee Indian who developed an alphabet for the Cherokee language and supposedly was able to teach his people to read in a matter of days, not years, he was interested in seeing the trees that he was named after.

So we dropped down from I-80 to go find a good route to Southern California and the Giant Redwoods. When we got to Las Vegas we stopped at a Mom and Pop grocery store and asked for directions. One of the customers who was purchasing a cheap bottle of wine volunteered to direct us.

"You go down here to the second intersection and turn right and go into prrrrrmmmmmmfmfmfmf."

"Where did you say?" I asked.

"purrr RUMMMM-ffff!

That was a lot clearer. Little did I know then that the man was telling the truth. There is town called Parumph. I thought he was drunk. But since the owner nodded his head in agreement with the customer, we bought some more pop and tried his directions. We had plenty of time. The worst that could happen is that we might get lost and lose a couple hours of time. We were almost two days ahead of schedule, so we weren't worried.

We should have been. Just as we got to the end of the long slow rise on this lonely county road, our transmission fluid boiled over. You can't drive very far when the automatic transmission fluid is gone. You can't drive period. So there we were halfway between Las Vegas and Parumph without a house in sight. Nothing but desert!

So Bob pulled out the tow rope in hopes that eventually somebody might come by and might offer to help us. Well, we might just as well attach it now to our car. So, Bob did and then returned to the driver's seat. Strictly for the hell of it, I picked up the other end of the tow rope to see if I could pull it. I could. It was ever so gentle a downhill grade. So, I decided we might have a better chance of someone stopping if they saw this old clown pulling the car.

Who knows if I was right. All I know is that after about a half hour, along came a woman my age driving a pickup truck. She told us that there was a service station right on the outskirts of Parumph that could help us, and she would give us a tow. She apologized that she wouldn't be able to drive very fast on account of her truck had something or other wrong with it. I can't remember exactly what. Neither can Bob. But we can both remember just how slow she drove.

Bob was behind the wheel, so I got in on the passenger side after tying the other end of our 12 foot tow rope to her towing bar. That left us about ten feet between the back of her truck and the front of our car. She started out very slowly so as not to snap the rope. That was nice. But then we watched the speedometer needle climb: 15, 20, 25, 30, 35. Yeah, 35 is a nice safe speed. Whoops, 40, 45. We began to get a bit uneasy. 50, 55, 60, 65, 70! There she held it. Bob and I both prayed that she wouldn't brake for a jackrabbit. There were two bumper stickers on the back of her pickup. One said, "I bought this in downtown Parumph." The other said, "I brake for animals."

Bob's eyes were glued on her taillights. I was praying. Thank God there were no curves along that road. Thank God that she merely tapped her brakes to signal she was going to slow down. She let Bob do the braking for her. Once we were there and unhooked, our gallant lady who towed us in wished us a good day and spun off. We went inside to get the transmission fluid.

Bob, always the boy scout, was prepared. He knew exactly how much we needed—five little half-pints. He spotted them and took them over to the cash register where a cute girl that Bob thought could make a cover girl was smiling at him. The five little half-pints were clearly marked $1.10 each. We both reached into our pockets to see if we had two quarters to go with the $5.00 bill I had pulled out of my wallet. And then both of us stared at what that beautiful young girl was doing.

She had taken out a pad of paper and carefully wrote down:

$$
\begin{array}{r}
1.10 \\
1.10 \\
1.10 \\
1.10 \\
+\ 1.10 \\
\end{array}
$$

Yes, she even wrote the plus sign down. Then she very carefully with her pencil went to the top of the right hand column and added all the zeros. And then put down a zero under the five zeros.

I looked at Bob. Bob looked at me. We didn't say a word. We just had to know what she would do next. Then she took pencil to the top of the next column and added each and every one. We could read her lips as she was saying to herself 1 plus 1 is 2 plus 1 is three plus another 1 is four and another 1 is 5! She wrote the five down. Then very carefully put the decimal point in before she added up the last column of 1's. And wonder upon wonders, she came up with 5, one more time.

"That will be $5.50, please." She was so pleasant to look at. Such a pleasant voice. But...that's not quite the end to that story. You see, later on that year I was in San Antonio at another convention and had struck up a conversation with a man who said he was from Las Vegas. So naturally I had to relate that story to him. He didn't believe that he would ever meet someone who had ever been to his hometown, Parumph. He had just said Las Vegas because nobody, not nobody, has ever heard of Parumph. As far as the girl is concerned. He knew exactly who she was. And she wasn't the class idiot. Far from it. He felt that Parumph had absolutely the worst teachers in the United States. Well, hopefully that isn't the case anymore because Parumph certainly has had time to improve their schools since 1976 when Bob and I were there.

Bob and I traveled all over. At least twice, we even took my daughter Linda with us. Once was to Concordia College in Moorhead, Minnesota where Linda was first exposed to the three magic words *cognitive*, *mastery*, and *automaticity* as the three phases in learning to read or spell. Those words tickled her funnybone.

Professor Downing used them over and over again while giving his series of lectures. And while Linda was amused by the words *cognitive*, *mastery* and *automaticity*, I had to admit there was more than just a little bit of truth to what he was saying. People can be presented with something and know it, sort of. For example, if I tell you that the sound of the word *sheep* is spelled шип in Russian. You know it for the moment. That kind of knowledge Professor Downing called *cognitive*. You kind of know it. If I worked with you for a few hours teaching you the sounds of a few more letters as in the chart below, you would be able to answer the questions after the chart on the next page correctly.

English letters	p	=	Russian letters	п
	ee	=		и
	sh	=		ш
	she	=		ши
	eep	=		ип
	sheep	=		шип
	keep	=		кип
	d	=		д
	k	=		к
	s	=		с

The correct spelling of the word **deep** using the Russian alphabet is: a— кир, b— дир, c— дип, d— пир

If you want to understand what *cognitive* means, look at the chart and figure out which word has to be the correct spelling of deep. That type of knowlege is very temporary. You can get the right answer. But how long can you maintain that knowledge necessary to pick out дип as being the spelling of deep?

If we worked on those letters for several days using a few multi-sensory techniques, that is:

- seeing the letters while hearing their sound
- saying the letters while seeing them and hearing their sound,
- writing the letters while seeing them and hearing their sound
- seeing the letters being written and being flashed while hearing them said separately and in combination with other letters and writing them,

you would be able to answer the question under that chart with ease. That would be the state of *mastery*.

If we worked on those letters and used them and used them so that you could read those words twenty-five years from now without hesitation, that is *automaticity*.

As much as Linda could understand the Professor Downing's concepts of *cognitive*, *mastery*, and *automaticity*, she still would giggle everytime she heard the words. Her attitude was that you didn't need to dress up common sense with words that just don't go together. *Cognitive* is unnecessarily academic. *Mastery* is a simple word whose meaning is changed to "you think you know it but you really don't." And *automaticity* is an invented word. It's not in any normal dictionary. Why use it? Well, I hated to admit to Linda that I thought she was right. So I didn't.

Our trip to Boise, Idaho to where I spoke at the Reading Reform Foundation's conference as well as exhibiting, was a different kind of trip. Bob made sure that the car was tuned up and that the tires were in good shape. We took turns driving the Chevette while Linda sat in the back supposedly navigating but mostly napping. As usual we left early giving ourselves plenty of time to visit tourist traps on the way to Idaho. That's why we took the very scenic route, crossing the Mackinac Bridge connecting the two peninulas of Michigan.

As as we were going through Wisconsin we found that we couldn't possibly speed even if we wanted to. Sensing that something might be wrong, we stopped at a Chevrolet dealership in Ashland. They couldn't find a thing wrong. So on we went. By the time we hit the bad lands our top speed was 50 miles per hour. When we reached Sydney, Montana, our top speed was 47 mph. We stopped there to visit my Aunt Esther and Uncle Leo. After an afternoon and evening of catching up on family affairs we were ready to go, but not before Uncle Leo took us over to the Chevrolet dealership where the service manager was a personal friend of his. Our Chevette got a free thorough check up. And passed with flying colors even though its top speed was only 47mph. The service manager thought it might have something to do with the altitude and the factory installed carburetor setting which he couldn't touch. So on we went. Just outside Billings, Linda decided we ought to drop down and visit Yellowstone National Park. Great idea. Except. Our top speed now was only 45 mph. We dropped down on highway 212 headed for Bear Tooth Pass where the altitude was almost 11,000 feet. As we headed up the mountain, our top speed kept dropping. When it got down to 30 mph, I was concerned. But Linda thought we could make it. By about 2:30 in the morning we were just a few miles from the top of the pass when the Chevette's speed was less than walking speed. Bob got out and thought he might help. But it wasn't long after before our top forward speed was zero. No matter how much I tried to race the motor, it wouldn't go forward. So, we turned it around and after a brief snowball fight, we got back in the car and drove down the mountain pass back toward Billings. It was about 3:00 in the morning when we tried to go through Red Lodge at top speed. A Red Lodge policeman with flashing lights pulled us over for speeding. We were clocked at 29 mph going through town where the speed limit was 25.

The policeman couldn't understand at first why Linda and Bob were laughing hysterically. I admitted to driving the Chevette at the fastest possible speed because I was afraid it would stall before we could get back to Billings where we hoped to find another Chevrolet dealership. I even offered him the opportunity to see if he could get the car up over 30 mph. He declined my offer. He even declined to issue us the speed ticket which he had intended to give us when he caught us in the Red Lodge speed trap.

When the dealership in Billings opened later that morning, we were there. Again, they couldn't find a thing wrong. So, on we went. The power was definitely lacking. If we were going down hill, we could get the car up to 50 mph now, but going up any sort of a grade, our top speed was 25. By the time we reached Boise, our top speed was 15 mph. The conference lasted only a couple days and then we started back. At the first gas station we stopped at, or rather hobbled into, the attendant told us that our problem was the catalytic converter being plugged. According to him, we must have picked up some leaded gas somewhere along the line. He told me that it wasn't uncommon in some areas to sell the cheaper leaded gas as unleaded to people passing through. He would have taken off the converter for us, but there were no tools at this service station. They only sold gas and oil. So we limped into Pocatello with our emergency lights flashing and driving mostly along the shoulder. At the Chevrolet dealership, I told him that the catalytic converter was plugged. He didn't think so. We had only 30,000 miles on the Chevette. It couldn't be plugged. Besides, they didn't have any catalytic converters in stock. They would have to order one, and it would take probably three or four days to get one. I asked him to at least remove the old plugged catalytic converter. He couldn't do it. It was against the law, he said. So, I asked him if it would be against the law to examine the converter. He guessed he could do that. In the meantime, he allowed me to talk to a salesman, who let me test drive a new car. That was nice of him. When I got back from the test drive, he showed me the converter. It was hopelessly plugged. Now, he had a problem. He couldn't just put it back on the way it was. He didn't have a replacement. So I asked him to just clean it out and put it back on. That he did, reluctantly. And off we drove. Once the obstruction in the exhaust system was eliminated, the Chevette drove just like new again.

We exhibited all over the United States, but we found out the hard way that most teachers are not interested in looking at materials being sold by a company they have never heard of. For the most part, teachers, administrators, and consultants attending conferences don't want to have their precious viewing time of the exhibits used up listening to any kind of sales pitch. And any explanation of the AVKO techniques, which were absolutely unknown to them, would be construed as a sales pitch. The most discouraging aspect of exhibiting was the way those with speaker's badges, those with badges that indicated that they were college instructors, or those with badges that indicated they were officers within whichever organization was holding the exhibit, the way these people would walk quickly by the AVKO exhibit without giving it a glance that would last over one second.

It's hard not to be paranoid. But almost any introduction to psychology instructor (or student) should be able to give the reason why. These people, the speakers, the college instructors, and the officers cannot afford to expose their ignorance. After all, they are the leaders. They keep up to date. They read all the important journals. If they haven't encountered studies about AVKO there, AVKO can't be important. Why waste their time? They have nothing to gain.

They might be embarrassed if they didn't understand what the Sequential Spelling technique was. It was easier for them to just pass by our exhibit.

But, I don't normally give up too easily. Okay, I'm stubborn. But I'm also somewhat flexible. I tried the inservice approach. Most schools have inservice days. Many schools just want to get the cheapest speaker possible for their teachers. So AVKO advertised me as an inservice speaker.

The most disappointing inservice that I ever put on was one in which I traveled to Wisconsin to put on an inservice for a group of parochial schools. I had asked them to bring students of all grade levels who had severe spelling problems, and I would demonstrate to them the AVKO Sequential Spelling technique.

They did provide the students. There were twenty students from grades three through nine. Not one could correctly spell the word *scattered* on the sheet of paper I had given them. So far so good. Then I began my magic.[1] I led them through the logical steps building from the *at* sound as in *bat* and *mat* and *flat* and *scat* to *batter* and *matter* and *flatter* and eventually *scattered*. As I was demonstrating the Sequential Spelling technique, I was explaining why it works. The teachers nodded their heads. They seemed to understand. When I was through we collected the students' papers. The result? Every single student correctly spelled the word *scattered*. Impressive? You would think so. But with teachers and school administrators, seeing isn't always believing and believing isn't always buying. The net result was that I sold one *AVKO Sequential Spelling I* book for $10.00. It had cost me $50.00 in gas and $80.00 for two nights in motels. I was a slow learner. I gave many a free inservice before deciding that this just didn't work.

Perhaps the most interesting inservice that I gave for which I was paid, was one that took place at Labette Community College in

---

[1]In chapter 19 I cover the exact technique that I used.

Parsons, Kansas. I was asked by Vivian Metcalf, the director of their reading center, to be the main speaker for what has since become an annual conference on dyslexia. This was their second one. She had somewhere encountered a brochure I had written called the AVKO challenge. In it, I stated that if I could not get the dyslexic of their choice to read the word *malicious* the first time I presented the word to the dyslexic to read, AVKO would pay for my fees and expenses. Otherwise, they would pay my speaker's fee and travel expenses. I also gave the same promise in reference to younger dyslexics and the spelling of the word *scattered*.

Most of the participants gave me very high marks on the presentation. They were genuinely impressed when I got four young men to spell the word *scattered* correctly after the audience found out they couldn't come close to correctly spelling it in the quick one sentence pretest.

They also were impressed with the adult dyslexic who did correctly read the word *malicious* the first time the adult dyslexic was asked to read it. But they had to take the word of the head of the clinic. The adult dyslexic was there anonymously and didn't want anyone to know who she was.

Afterwards, I casually asked the director of the Learning Center who the adult dyslexic was. She smiled and said, "Joyce Hochanadel, the president's wife. Three of the four boys you worked with are sons of staff members here at the college."

Now, it was apparent to me that they wanted me for my approach as a means to helping specific individuals. Theory is fine, but results are better. They got their results. The last I knew, the dyslexics who performed for me had someone using AVKO materials and techniques with them and have become adequate readers and spellers.

So, we decided to forget about promoting sales and to concentrate on developing materials and techniques and to work almost exclusively with dyslexics at the Foundation.

Part III
Educational Research: In what direction/s should AVKO go?

Chapter 15

FREE *DAILY* Tutoring at the AVKO Foundation's Reading Clinic.

AVKO HAS NEVER WIDELY advertised that it offers free DAILY tutoring at the AVKO Reading Clinic. But when people would call or visit the foundation, we have never turned anyone away. But notice that we put the emphasis on *daily*. There are a number of good reasons for the emphasis upon DAILY.

- If someone isn't learning to read (and/or spell) while going to school six hours a day, thirty hours a week, what kind of magic hocus pocus will it take to do in two hours a week what the school can't do in thirty hours.

- Tutoring, to be truly effective, must be on a daily basis.

- Standard tutoring rates are $30.00 an hour. This is what ordinary certified teachers charge. This would mean that if I were to charge the going rate and have my students for one hour five days a week, I would have to charge them $150.00. That's a lot money for most folks.

- But what *should* I charge *if* I were to charge? Shouldn't it be considerably more than the average? If an ordinary run-of-the-mill lawyer charges $70.00 an hour and a good lawyer $700.00 an hour, how much more should I?

- How many reading tutors do you know who are listed in *Who's Who*? How many reading tutors do you know who are listed in *The Yearbook of Experts, Authorities, & Spokespersons*? How many reading tutors have written books?

- Learning reading and spelling takes time. Even advancing students at the rate of 1 year in reading level every two months, it would take approximately 14 months or $2,100.00 to bring most older students up to snuff. And who can afford that much? The rich can, I know. They do spend that. And more!

- But should AVKO cater only to the rich? Our answer was no.

- Rather than charge a token amount that could be interpreted as being what our lessons are worth, we decided not to charge anything except for materials. But what we are doing isn't that much different than what Clarence Darrow did in real life in the legal field. He took on many *pro bono* cases. And all that legalese just means, "it's free—for the good."

One of our first live-in students was a young man from Indiana whose name really was exactly the same as one of the more famous names in the Phonics-is-Bad school of thought. We'll call him Kenny Goodman. He was about fifteen and he still couldn't read and write. His mother was at her wits' end.

She had taken him everywhere to be tested. At least everywhere she knew to take him within driving distance of her home—and that included Indiana University. She was told by everyone who tested him, that her Ken Goodman couldn't be taught.

Then someone told her about AVKO. She called and talked to me on the phone. After I heard her story, I made the very brash statement, that indeed Kenny could be taught to read at least as well as he can speak. However, I told her that if the experts said he couldn't be taught, that means to me that I won't be able to teach him to read in just one hour a day. I would have to have complete control over everything he does all day long. In other words, he would have to stay at the foundation.

I could hear her gulp. "How much would that cost?"

Room and board and materials. We don't charge for testing and tutoring. Her sigh of relief was audible.

"Are you sure you can teach Kenny?" she asked.

I told her that I was sure enough that if I couldn't get him to read or to spell the word *scattered* the first time I gave it to him or read the word *malicious* the first time I showed it to him (her choice), the AVKO Foundation would reimburse her for her travel expenses up here.

She chose to see if Ken could learn to spell the word *scattered* without ever having seen the word. For extra verification of the effectiveness of the technique I use, I asked Kenny's mother to have him attempt to spell the word for her and to bring a copy of his misspelling of the word with them when they came.

She brought him up on the next Sunday. Kenny's misspelling of the word *scattered* was *sadr*. Needless to say when I went through my little snake oil routine, Kenny correctly spelled *scattered*! So she left him with me for eight weeks.

When she left, I warned her that Kenny might be an entirely different young man when she next saw him. I was right. And it's a good thing I was right. At the time he came to AVKO, Kenny exhibited what I call the "whipped dog" syndrome. He was completely lacking in self-confidence and self-esteem. He walked stiffly and slowly with his head and shoulders drooping down. What had happened to him in school, I could only speculate. I didn't want to know, and I never asked. Let bad memories like sleeping dogs lie quietly. Ken's days began with exercise. I taught to him to throw and catch a ball, to ride a bicycle. I worked on his reading and his spelling. We used my materials and lots of other materials including my favorite Dr. Seuss books. Ken learned to make his bed, clean his room, cook and do dishes (when it was his turn) and to operate the washer and drier. Kenny is now living independently somewhere in Indiana. We still keep in touch.

Among the large number of students who have come to the AVKO Reading Clinic for help, no one was more challenging than Norman Menninger. He had been in Special Education all through school. He graduated unable to read anything except for a few scattered words considered by his teachers to be essential and a few scattered words he considered to be essential. For example, Norman could read *BAR* but couldn't read *bar* or *Bar*. Why? You guessed it. Signs advertising a place where he could get a beer were important to him. But notice that the appearance of each letter in ***BAR*** is entirely different than in ***bar***. Norman was responding to a picture-graphic not to letters. I wish that I could say that Norman was a success story. He wasn't. But he could have been. The State of Michigan hired a blind man to test Norman. Based on the results of his tests (which were not made available to AVKO) this blind man insisted that no attempt should be made to get Norman to respond to phonic patterns. The blind man also used a pre- and post testing device that neither measures gains correctly or diagnoses correctly. The State of Michigan also demanded great improvement in three months. Well, the blind man's tests didn't indicate a great enough gain and the state withdrew its support which really only paid for Norman's room and board.

But Norman taught me one thing. And that is when the philosophies of Frank Smith, Ken Goodman, and the other leading whole language gurus are taken to extremes, the results can be amusing. For example, whenever Norman encountered WATCH he read BEWARE. If the sentence was TOM GAVE MARY A WATCH FOR CHRISTMAS. Norman would read TOM GAVE MARY A BEWARE FOR CHRISTMAS. The only explanation I have for that is that he was taught to read road signs. WATCH FOR ICE ON BRIDGE. This meant BEWARE of ice. He had locked in a meaning and not sound plus meaning with that five letter combination.

I have had many who when they came to me would read the word *house* as *pony* as in, "She opened the door and walked into the *pony!*" The words *horse* and *house* look so much alike that it is easy for the "picture-graphic" to have a meaning and a sound attached to it that has no bearing on the actual letters in the word. For example, many a well meaning teacher has refused to correct a student when he read "Mary wanted to ride her horse to school," as "Mary wanted to ride her pony to school." The concept of reading being a psycholinguistic guessing game allows its true believers to rarely correct the student. Sometimes (not always obviously) the student attaches the sound and meaning of *__pony__* to the letters h-o-r-s-e. And if the sound and meaning of the word *__house__* is attached to the letter h-o-m-e, then the picture-graphic of *__house__* can easily be mistaken for the picture-graphic of *__horse__* which is *__pony__* to the Norman Menningers of this world.

Another thing about Norman that I discovered to be true of many illiterates. They don't sing. Not even a note. I tried to use music with Norman as a tool. But Norman said he could not sing, and he would not sing one single word. Since his mother was a choir director at the church he attended, I jumped to the two-bit psychological conclusion, that if Norman didn't sing he couldn't be yelled at for being either off-key or for singing the wrong word.

One of the more interesting dyslexics who came to the AVKO Clinic for free daily tutoring was Brian Nagurski who lived in a little town called Fostoria about twenty-five miles away. Every morning he was dropped off by his parents who ran a printing business in Flint. And every evening he was picked up. Brian had graduated from his high school at the very bottom of his class. He wanted to join the U.S. Marine Corps, but he was told he would have to learn to read before he could even think about taking the test. Becoming a marine was his motivation. One of the many techniques I used with Brian was reading the funnies. The moment his parents dropped him off, he was responsible for bringing in the morning paper, *The Detroit Free Press.* He had to attempt to read at least Peanuts and Calvin. Calvin was a trip. But Brian didn't want to be the only one not in on the jokes. If he couldn't read a word, he asked, and he got the help he needed. He used the AVKO Individualized Keyboarding program and learned to type as well as locking in phonic patterns and spellings of words. He was a good student. He learned. After ten months, he just knew he would pass the test to enter the Marine Corps. And pass it he did. With flying colors. Unfortunately, Brian never was able to become a U.S. Marine. Just before he was scheduled to take his physical, he tried running off the end of a dock and catching a football just like one of the stunt men in the Mountain Dew commercials that were all over the TV that year. Only unlike the commercial, his ending was not very graceful. He came down on the edge of the dock and severed his achilles tendon. So, instead of becoming a Marine, he became a college student. He's probably one of the very few college graduates who was the very last in his high school graduating class.

Every summer AVKO has had kids coming for the free daily tutoring. And each year, they seemed to be coming from a different town. One year they were from Montrose. Another, from St. Charles or Clio. Or Mt. Morris, Millington, or Birch Run. And even from Houston, Texas as did Philip Bergman.

I first met Philip Bergman at an Orton Dyslexia Society conference where his father was promoting "The Bridge." This was a computer program developed for the Atari computer, which Philip's father, Dr. Eldo Bergman, thought would be within the means of most families or school systems to purchase for dyslexics.

Dr. Bergman showed me how his computer program worked. I showed him the AVKO materials and the basic AVKO approach. I think he thought AVKO's materials seemed almost too good to be true. He liked what he saw. He liked what he heard. But still, would it work for his son Philip?

Dr. Bergman, who quickly let me know he wanted to be called simply by his nickname Skip, told me that Philip who was in high school at the time, had received every traditional treatment for dyslexia. Skip, who is a pediatric neurologist, told me that he and his wife, who is a pediatrician, had noticed in the first grade that Philip wasn't learning to read. They had him tested. There was no question about it. Philip was a bright young boy with a very high I.Q., but he wasn't learning to read. He was a dyslexic.

So since the public school didn't have a special program for dyslexic youngsters, the Bergmans put Philip in a private school where the maximum classroom load was six. You would think that this would have really helped Philip. He entered the private school in the second grade reading at a 1.7 grade level. After two years of the private school, Philip tested out at 1.9. Two months gain in two years of private school didn't satisfy either of the two Doctor Bergmans.

So they hired a private tutor who was a follower or true believer of the Rudolph Flesch school of thought that the reason *Why Johnny Can't Read* is that he hasn't been taught phonics intensively. It did help some. One year of private tutoring with heavy, heavy phonics Philip went from a reading level of 1.8 to 2.8, but by now he had finished the fourth grade. So now Philip was sent for tutoring to a reading specialist recommended by the local Orton Dyslexia Society which used the Orton-Gillingham multi-sensory approach and more phonics. For the next four years Philip had this Alpha-Betic Phonics approach used. And he *was* improving his reading. But not rapidly at all. In fact, he was gaining only a half year in reading skills for a whole year of special tutoring. That was when Skip developed his computer program to help his son write compositions. And from that time forward, Philip was steadily progressing. By the time Philip was going into the 11th grade, he was now reading at the 6.5 grade level as measured by the Woodcock Johnson test. His reading speed was slow. With material written at a 4th grade level, Philip's silent reading speed was barely 60 words per minute. And when you consider that people speak at double that rate, you know something is seriously wrong.

Philip's spelling was something else. It was *troole fonek* (truly phonic). Or at least it was according to the way he had been taught. When I told Skip that I could get Philip to correctly spell either the word *scattered* or the word *malicious* the first time I gave it to him and without him once seeing, hearing, or writing the correct spelling, Skip was very skeptical. But he patronized me. To protect his son from embarrassment, he let me go for the word *scattered*. Skip was amazed at how quickly I got Philip to correctly spell the word. So, he accepted the AVKO challenge and invited me to speak in Houston before a group of parents, dyslexics, and the head of the special education department of the Houston schools.

I spoke and I demonstrated. All the younger kids correctly learned to spell the word *scattered*. The older kids? I got them to correctly spell *malicious*. That convinced Skip that I could really help Philip. It also convinced another mother of an older boy named Matt Henderson, that he could learn from me. So, arrangements were made for the two boys to come to the AVKO Foundation for six weeks of free tutoring. They only paid for room and board and miscellaneous expenses.

In six weeks Philip's reading level jumped from 6.5 to 9.5. His reading speed went from 60 to over 200 words per minute. Matt Henderson made even more spectacular gains.

How is that possible? Well, if AVKO believed only in using one set of techniques, it certainly wouldn't be possible. The spectacular gains were the result of a combination of factors. One, both Philip and Matt were well motivated. They both knew that they were intelligent. They both knew that their failure to learn to read was not their fault. They both knew that I knew my business. I knew words. I knew spelling. I knew how to teach. They expected to learn. Oh, the power of expectancy! If kids expect to learn, they usually do. If kids expect that nothing can help them, nothing can.

Of the many techniques I used with them, the one that I think helped Matt the most, was my Adult Phonics Folders. These are regular manilla folders. I had a separate folder for each Adult Phonic Pattern. The folder marked -cious had in it about a hundred different colorful magazine ads. Each of the ads had one *-cious* word highlighted. For example, one was an ad for a popular beverage with the word *delicious* highlighted. Another was an ad from a medical magazine advertising a mood altering drug. It showed a picture of an elderly woman scowling. The word highlighted was *suspicious*. As you can imagine there were many ads using the word *delicious* and *vivacious* and *spacious* and *vicious* and even *malicious*.

The way we used them wasn't really any different from the standard way flash cards are used. But our ads had several advantages over standard flash cards. First of all, they had pictures and graphics and were attractive to the eye and they were from ADULT magazines such as *Better Homes and Gardens, Ebony, People, Popular Mechanics, Time,* etc.—not kiddy stuff. But more importantly, the highlighted -cious words were in different sizes and styles of print. Some were all in UPPER CASE; others all in lower.

Without them realizing it, by going through these little drills, their eyes were being trained to scan. Their minds were being trained to react rapidly and swiftly to patterns and to words.

Not all AVKO's students made such great gains in such a short space of time. We had one from Pennsylvania, who like Brian Nagurski, wanted to pass the Army's entrance examination. But he wasn't willing to spend the time we told him would be necessary. He wanted to be able to pass the test after six weeks of intensive tutoring. We tried. He made very good gains. But, it wasn't just enough to be able to read the questions to pass the test. John Stakowski had never really wanted to learn much of anything. He boasted to us about how he used to roam the halls and shake down other students in the lavatories. He didn't know his multiplication tables, nor did he want to. Forget about simple arithmetic. He could care less. He knew what he wanted out of life. Lots of women, plenty of booze and a big pay check. Although he agreed to pay for his room and board, he managed to leave owing us over $200.00 for his food and a telephone bill for 900 numbers he called to listen to pornographic talk of over $300.00. He skipped out. After that sad experience we reluctantly adopted the standard practice of asking for the first and last month's payments in advance. And what happened to John Stakowski? The last we knew, he didn't pass his test. But he didn't come back.

But John Stakowski wasn't the only ungrateful student we have had who has taken advantage of our offers of free tutoring. The most outstanding and recent example of ingratitude is that of a wealthy Danish newspaper owner and his dyslexic daughter. Because AVKO is listed in many standard reference tools used by librarians all over the world, he got our number from a library in Copenhagen. He called us and asked for help for his daughter. He wanted his daughter Carmen to spend a year in the United States attending a college as he had done when he was 18. The problem was that she was dyslexic and wanted to study art. He wanted us to try to find a place, preferably in Michigan, where she could study art and receive help for her dyslexia.

I gave him the name of the Orton Dyslexia Society to contact, as they specialize in helping parents find help for their students. I also called the major universities in Michigan and talked with a counselor at each of them. I did not receive much encouragement. But I did check out Mott Community College in Flint and the University of Michigan Flint Campus. What I found out is that if Carmen were to attend the University of Michigan her tuition would be $10,000 a year and her freshman art instructors would be the same identical instructors teaching at Mott Community College. The two schools were sharing the same facilities and instructors! Mott's tuition for a foreign student was based on credit hours taken and came out to being over $6,000.00 less than U of M Flint.

I let him know about Mott and their program and the limited services they had for dyslexics. I told him that neither school provided dormitories. I also told him that AVKO did provide free daily tutoring. If Carmen wanted to study art at Mott, we would help her by providing a place to stay (room and board at $100.00 a week) and an automobile to use free except for gas, oil, incidental repairs, and insurance which we estimated to be only around $50.00 a month because it was being shared by another student. Guess who? Philip Bergman, back after a two year hiatus, for more free tutoring from the foundation while he studies art at Mott. Carmen's father thought that this would be a great opportunity for her—and a great savings for him.

So after many faxes and letters and trips to Mott Community College and talking to counselors and the head of the art department, Carmen was accepted.

Carmen was to arrive at the Flint Bishop International Airport in the evening on the 7:30 flight from Detroit. My wife and I got there early because on occasion the twenty minute flight from Detroit got there early. And it did. At 7:20 the passengers got off. But no Carmen. Back to the the airline ticket counter. Check, check, check. Finally, the clerk discovered on her computer that Carmen had missed her connecting flight. Although she had plenty of time to go from one gate to the other, she took her time. She missed her flight. So we had to wait until 11:30 for her. She was happy that we were there to greet her. But she expected no less. She didn't bother to thank us. As I would discover later, the words, "Thank you," rarely crossed her lips.

We stopped at a restaurant on the way back and bought her a meal. Not a thank you. But a lot of complaints about the service and the airlines. We brought her to the foundation and showed Carmen her room, a rather spacious 12 x 15 room with large closets and 12 feet of counter space and a six foot drawing table. She got up fourteen hours later. Although her father said she knew how to drive and had taken driving lessons and had an international drivers license, I didn't just give her directions on how to get to Mott Community College. I went with her. She drove. Oh, did she drive! I almost had a heart attack. And her sense of direction was absolutely non-existent. She missed turns. She didn't know what to do if she passed a street that she was supposed to make a right hand turn on. One time she drove five miles after being told she missed her turn before she finally found a driveway to turn into. Then when she returned the five miles she made a right hand turn. Apparently she didn't understand that to go the right direction, in this case west, if you're driving south you make a right hand turn. If you miss it and return, you are now driving north. If you make a right hand turn now, you're driving east.

Carmen was not ready to drive in the streets of Flint, Michigan and its crazy expressways. She wasn't ready really to drive anywhere. So now, if Carmen was to be able to go to and from Mott College she would have to take driving lessons. She couldn't (or wouldn't) afford a driving school. Besides, her classes were scheduled to start in ten days. So guess who was elected to teach her? Moi!

When Philip arrived I discovered that he, too, knew little or nothing about driving. He had no license. So, I had to get him a permit and teach him to drive. But at this, Philip was a fast learner. And I thanked God that he was one dyslexic who had a sense of direction. As long as he was in the car, I knew that Carmen couldn't get lost.

Although Carmen could speak English well enough to communicate her needs, no one ever really knew whether she understood anything we said to her. And that really posed a major problem at the AVKO reading clinic and at Mott. Her reading level couldn't really be measured by any standardized test as being above 1.0. For all intents and purposes, she could not read a word of English nor could she spell anything other than her name.

She had a certified check for $14,000.00 to deposit plus another check for some rather large amount but unknown to me. The trip to the bank was a trip and a half. I knew she would have to have all her identification papers with her when she went. Before we left, I reminded her and asked her if she had them. She smiled and said, "Yes." When we got there and began the procedures, she was asked for her passport. She didn't have it with her. Back to the AVKO Clinic. Back to the bank. Now she was asked for her student papers. Back to the AVKO Clinic. Back to the bank. The woman who was the branch manager tried to communicate with her. It was tough. But I helped Carmen understand that a savings account would bring her interest, would make some money for her while a checking account would cost her money in bank charges. She elected to have two savings accounts. One just for her personal money and one for the money given to her from her father.

I walked her through the registration process and saved her the expense of having to wait in long lines. It just so happened that one of the counselors was an old buddy of mine from Flint Tech, Dan Stetz. He cut through loads of red tape and signed up Carmen for her classes. He even helped convince the school that Carmen shouldn't be forced to take the requisite English classes and that her studies at the AVKO clinic along with the nine credit hours at Mott would satisfy the U.S. Immigration's requirement that she be a full time (i.e., 12 credit hour student). The difference was also a $273.00 savings for her.

With Philip guiding her and taking two of the same classes, Carmen was able to get through the first semester with no major problems, except that she just didn't think it necessary to get all her immigration papers completely filled out and signed by the school. Three times she was called into the office. Three times she promised to get the papers and bring them in, but she never did.

Christmas vacation came. Carmen decided to fly to Edmonton, to visit a girl friend from Denmark who was an exchange student staying with a Canadian family. The morning of her flight, she asked Philip to drive her to the airport. From my bedroom I could hear the car start up, and it sounded bad. When Philip returned it sounded worse. It sounded like it was about to throw a rod. The Toyota, which had been donated to AVKO, was worth about $1,200.00 as long as it could run. But to replace the engine would be more than $1,200.00. We had it towed to a rarity, an absolutely honest mechanic. He told us that the engine was beyond repair. In his opinion, the motor had been running without enough oil for some period of time. It was only then that I discovered that Philip had only once bothered to check the oil when he filled the tank. Carmen, never. And I had given both Carmen and Philip instructions to do just that and had explained the reason why.

Carmen was scheduled to come back on December 29th. But she didn't. She was being held back by the immigration officials because she didn't have the papers signed by Mott Community College verifying that she was enrolled full time. Poor Angela Reeves. She was at a holiday party when the school tracked her down for Carmen. Angela had to leave the party, get special papers signed for Carmen, and have them sent Federal Express overnight to Edmonton.

But was AVKO informed by Carmen that she wasn't coming? No. When she finally got her papers and clearance to return, did she call? No. I got the information from the man who had been gracious enough to let her visit her friend who was staying with them. From talking to him, I got the clear impression that he thought Carmen expected everybody to do everything for her and let her have her own way about everything.

When Carmen arrived at the airport she was surprised to see Ann and me there. She had called her boy friend from Edmonton and had expected him to pick her up and take her to his house. She spoke not a single word on the trip from the airport back to the AVKO Foundation. She only grunted a few indistinguishable sounds when asked if she had a good time in Canada. So, we left it at that.

Carmen didn't get up the next morning. She didn't get up until 3:00 in the afternoon. I explained the situation about the Toyota. She grunted. Then she asked if she could drive into Flint! When I re-explained the situation she just said, "So? If it breaks down, it breaks down. That's none of your business. You don't have to worry about me."

I told her that her days of my being her personal chauffeur were over. She flounced out of the room. A few hours later she announced that she was going out on New Year's Eve and that her boy friend would pick her up. Fine. My wife asked her what time she expected to get back. "When I get back!" was her snarly answer.

Ann looked at me and sighed as if to say, "What's the use?"

Carmen got back sometime after 5:00 a.m. She got up at 4:00 p.m. At that point, I decided to have a serious discussion with her. I first asked her to write the names of people who have done nice things for her any time during the last year. After she compiled the list of names, I asked her to transfer the names one at a time on separate sheets of paper. I had her draw a line down the middle of each sheet. On the left hand side I asked her to list the nice things they did for her. She came back with the list all written in Danish. For some strange reason I didn't accept that. I asked her to write it in English. I would help her spell whatever word she needed.

Finally, the lists of nice things that each person did for her was completed. Then I asked her to write on the right hand side of each paper what nice things she did for all these different people. The best she could muster was that she had loaned some money to Philip, she had loaned some money to her girl friend, she had helped her boy friend with his homework in art class once, and she had loaned money to her girl friend in Canada. That was it. Well, not quite. On a number of the sheets, she had written, "I said thank you." But not on the sheet that bore my name. From the day she arrived to the day she left, not once did she thank me for anything. Maybe she considered me to be her servant since her daddy was paying for everything. And maybe in Denmark one doesn't ever say thank you to a servant. I don't know.

Then I went through a list of possible New Year's Resolutions which included such horrible things as being up at least by 10:00 every morning, having at least two lessons every day, and calling me by my correct name, Mr. McCabe. "Yes, Don." was her answer.

The next morning I had an appointment at McLaren Hospital in Flint to have a stress test taken. It had been three years since my heart attack and my physician felt I should have another test. When I left, I stopped by the Florist shop in the hospital and bought a nice flowering plant. I then went to Mott Community College and went directly to the office of Angela Reeves, thanked her for what she had done for Carmen and gave her the flowering plant as a token of appreciation.

Angela expressed to me her feelings about the foreign exchange students she had to deal with who came from Denmark. "Spoiled rotten" were her words. She also said that everything has to be their way, and that they have no concern for others. Harsh words. Then she thanked me.

When I got home, Carmen was packed ready to leave. Her boy friend was going to pick her up. I did manage to get her to sign a document saying she was leaving of her own free will. But even before that, I called her father. That she was leaving was news to him. He called her. She wouldn't listen to him. She was leaving and that was that.

And she did. Did she tell me where she was going? No. Did she ask us to forward her mail? No. She just took off. I had another long talk with her father, and he explained that he was in a logical bind. He had told Carmen that he had wanted to have her have the same experience that he had and to learn to make her own decisions. And when she made her own decisions, what could he say? She kept throwing his own words back at him. It was *her* decision to make—not his.

Since one of the perks of owning a major foreign newspaper happens to be covering major sporting events, Carmen's father was going to the Super Bowl in Minneapolis. After watching the San Francisco 49ers crush the San Diego Chargers, he came to Flint to see his daughter and to visit the AVKO Foundation. He seemed genuinely pleased to meet me and impressed with what he saw. He apologized for his daughter's behavior but again mentioned the fact that he was caught in a trap of his own making. He wanted his daughter to experience the United States and to make her own decisions. If she runs out of money, she runs out of money. He wasn't going to bail her out anymore than his own father bailed him out.

He took samples of the AVKO materials with him and left. Later I got a very flattering letter saying that he had sent my materials to a friend of his who was a university professor. At the end of the letter, almost like an afterthought, he asked for an accounting of Carmen's bills and payments with us.

That should have sent up a red flag. But dyslexics tend to be trusting souls. It hadn't occurred to me to ask why he didn't bring Carmen with him when he came to visit. I had thought that he just wanted to see the AVKO Foundation for himself and to be able to talk to me freely without Carmen being around to listen in. As I would later find out, he had asked Carmen to come with him, and she had refused saying she was afraid of me. Or was she afraid of being caught in lies? I believe the latter.

But anyway, I obliged him. I tallied the cost of the ruined Toyota for which we couldn't even find a used motor to be put in it. I divided it in two and charged Carmen for that and for her share of the insurance. Since I didn't have the facts in front of me, I asked the bookkeeper for a costing of the insurance. It was quite a bit more than just $50.00 a month, 209.08 to be exact. So, Carmen's share of the insurance and the repairs to make the auto safe for her were figured in. After all the figures were computed, we estimated that Carmen owed AVKO $514.00. We itemized everything and carefully explained each item and faxed him the bill that we intended to give to Carmen.

Explosion time! To Carmen's father I was a cheat. I had no right to bill Carmen for destroying the Toyota. That was my tough luck. I should have checked the oil myself. I should not have charged Carmen for the added insurance costs. I had agreed to $50.00 for the car to cover everything. If I had made a mistake or costs had gone up, that was my responsibility, not his. An agreement is an agreement! And I had no right to hold back the money that Carmen had given for the months of January and June. He wasn't going to let me cheat him or cheat Carmen out of one penny!

Reason and facts would not appease him. He would not answer any of my yes or no questions about what he wanted for Carmen. He didn't care how many thousands of dollars I may have saved him, he wasn't going to let me cheat him or Carmen out of anything.

Oh, well as it is often said, no good deed goes unpunished. Carmen left and never returned nor would she pay what she owed us. Nor would she or her father agree to third-party arbitration.

But Carmen wasn't the only ungrateful recipient of free daily tutoring. And probably won't be the last.

The oldest dyslexic that I worked with was Albert Dolan. Talk about an intelligent illiterate. This man learned to be a photographer and run his own darkroom. He became a union steward and handled grievances in the shop. He worked as a deputy sheriff. He runs his own landscaping business. And he couldn't read nor spell anything beyond his own name, and even that he misspelled. Well, not entirely. It's just that he never capitalized his first name. Albert Dolan could copy. He could fake it. His wife did all his reading for him. It wasn't until she developed a chronic debilitating disease that confined her to a wheel chair and prevented her from doing his reading and writing for him, that he finally sought help from AVKO. How did Al find out about AVKO? Well, his nephew was a golfing buddy of mine. And his nephew gave him my name. The rest is history.

Although the total number of people we have helped over the years isn't particularly impressive, the following happens to be true. Of the five nearest neighboring houses with children, at least one from each of the five families received help. The total of the neighborhood children who received help from AVKO was 8 out of a possible 10. Maybe there was something in the ground water! I even had to help my own son to read when he finished first grade unable to read.

One of our neighbors had a son who is an epileptic and who has a mild case of cerebral palsy. He was a special education student all his school life. When he graduated from high school he read at about the third grade level. Since that time he has received some help from the foundation. His reading level now is about at the seventh or eighth grade level. And he is a volunteer at the AVKO Foundation, running our copy machines, punching and binding, proofreading even, and all kinds of tasks. Willie Brown was and is grateful for the help we've given him. And he shows it with his volunteering.

On the other hand, we had two neighborhood boys whom we helped by not only giving them free tutoring but by giving them jobs at the foundation and working our Bingo. One was an athlete and bright and personality plus with the name of Maurice L'Amour. The other, Franklin L'Amour was a plodder, honest and sincere, but a hopeless klutz. Maurice repaid us for helping him by stealing over $2,000.00 from us. His own mother called and told us that he was the one. But he had destroyed the evidence (the AVKO briefcase and the AVKO Bingo records but not the cash) and the State Police didn't want to bother themselves with such a petty crime. Maurice ended up selling dope and running numbers. One of my neighbors told me that I got what I deserved for helping out them "niggers." But, Franklin tried to make something out of himself. Eventually he got a job as a security guard in Detroit and got himself killed. You just never can tell.

Part III, Chapter 16

The teaching of reading:
Religious cults in conflict.

ONE OF THE THINGS I tell nearly everybody who questions me about the AVKO approach, is that I am thankful that I learned how to teach reading and spelling before I took any education courses. If I had gotten a doctorate in reading at Michigan State University before I started teaching reading, it's quite possible that I would never have learned the simple truths. I might have been so filled with the latest theories and studies that I might have missed the obvious.

Don't get me wrong. I learned a lot from my instructors at Michigan State. Maybe not exactly what they wanted me to learn, but learn I did. When I applied for admission for my doctoral program in 1976, I deliberately set out to get the biggest names in reading on MSU's staff to be on my committee. Gerry Scruffy, the author of a book that preached systematic teaching of reading, seemed the logical choice. And he was. The problem is he was beginning to change his philosophy to coincide with the gurus of the whole language movement. And he wanted me to change my thinking, too. He was into what he called the *process* of instruction. And to give the man credit, he did his best to expose all his students to all the various schools of thought about the teaching of reading. Well, almost all. He certainly didn't expose his students to the AVKO concepts. He didn't mention Orton-Gillingham, Slingerland, or Schmerler. Phonics he dismissed as just a crutch to beginning reading. Commercial materials such as SRA Reading Laboratories were taboo even for discussion. But to give the man credit, he made sure I took courses from instructors who had differing points of view. At least they all had differing points of view than mine.

They all looked at reading as being a process that began before school started as part of verbal expression. But as far as they were concerned for academic study purposes, the process really ended around the third grade. The theory was once the process was fully started it kept going by itself. Their concerns were all centered around what ways were the best ways to get the process started.

What Dr. Scruffy objected to was my contention that any real solution to the widespread problem of functional illiteracy in the United States (and elsewhere) would only be found if the academic researchers made exhaustive studies on the following:

- What *specific words* can functional illiterates read.
- Were those specific words taught or encountered frequently?
- Were the phonic components of these words taught or encountered frequently.

And of course the converse follows, that a solution to the widespread problem of functional illiteracy would only be found if the academic researchers made exhaustive studies on the following:

- What specific words are functional illiterates unable to read.
- Were these specific words ever systematically taught? If so, what methods were used?
- Were the phonic components of these words systematically taught?
- If the phonic components of these specific words are systematically taught will the previously functionally illiterate be able to decode these specific words without them being specifically taught as units? For example, if students are taught -ci-=/sh/ and -ous=/us/ and that

cious=/shus/, will they be able to decode words
such as *gracious, precious,* and *malicious*?

Dr. Scruffy admitted it was an interesting concept, but never did he
pursue it in class or mention it to any of his students. Now, he also
knew that I was the Research Director of the AVKO Educational
Research Foundation, and that I was the author of a number of books
on reading and on spelling. But he never mentioned the fact to his
classes. And I thought it would be inappropriate for me to bring it up.
Actually, I should have been suspicious. Scruffy knew I wanted to get
my Ph.D. as soon as possible. He agreed with me that a Ph.D. behind
my name would be essential to get the academic community to listen
to my ideas. He knew I wanted to begin work on my thesis as soon
as possible. Despite this, he kept delaying calling a committee
meeting and wouldn't discuss possible topics for my dissertation with
me.

One class that I took from him was a class that not only spanned
two semesters but used two teachers. Dr. Scruffy was one. The other
was Dr. Molar. The first semester went rather uneventfully. Because
everyone was to receive a grade for both semesters only at the end of
the second semester, most of the students did not have all their
requisite papers completed at the end of the first semester. But I did.

A week before the end of the second semester we were covering
the topic "The Tools of Instruction." One student started out saying
something like "The quality of instruction may often depend upon the
quality of the tools being used." And as was the policy in his
classroom, if you wanted to address the point, you raised your hand
at that time and then later on Dr. Scruffy would call on you. I raised
my hand.

But almost immediately Dr. Scruffy interrupted the student and
launched into a rather long diatribe proclaiming that it was the
techniques that a teacher employed that brought about a learning

situation. Tools by themselves are unimportant. In this class we should concentrate on techniques not on tools.

After about ten minutes of this diatribe, Dr. Scruffy called on me. All I said was, "You've made it clear to me that you don't believe that the tools of instruction have any significance. So there's no point in me wasting your time and the class's time in pointing out how important the tools of instruction really are."

Dr. Scruffy became livid. He screamed at me, "McCabe, if you open your mouth one more time I'll physically throw you out of this class."

I didn't say another word to him. Nor did I return to the class. There wasn't any point in talking to Dr. Molar who witnessed Dr. Scruffy's violent reaction to me. Dr. Molar was his wife.

I received a letter from Dr. Scruffy saying that he would no longer be the chairperson of my doctoral committee nor would he serve on the committee in any capacity.

I did finally get Dr. Herman (who co-authored the text *Systematic Reading Instruction* with Dr. Scruffy) to take over as chairperson. By the way, no committee meeting had ever taken place. I had wanted one, but Dr. Scruffy had kept saying it wasn't time yet. He kept saying that we really didn't have to follow the normal procedures outlined in the manual. Those are just written rules because the department needs to have something written down. But they don't really mean a thing. Uh, huh. Naïve little dyslexic McCabe actually believed him.

Dr. Herman followed the same approach. Now, he was the one in charge of the special remedial reading clinic at Michigan State. Here children in the community with reading problems were diagnosed and tutored by graduate students. In his class, he assigned me a student he assured the class couldn't be taught to read. He had already been tested and assigned a tutor twice before. Since we were allowed to use any materials, I used my own, but in a very different way. Since the student came in for only 45 minutes and only twice a week, I knew then that I would have to do something different. That something different was to engage the help of his mother. I showed her how to use my Sequential Spelling with her son at home. Just ten minutes a day, but every single day—Sundays included.

I worked with him using fairly traditional techniques such as neurological impress. But don't be impressed with that term. All it really means is read-along-with-me. But instead of positioning myself behind him and have him follow my galloping finger, I sat directly across the corner from him and read with him upside down.

Dr. Herman who observed behind one-way glass was dumbfounded. Not only did I read upside down, but I wrote upside down! He had never seen a tutor ever do that before. So in the class discussion that generally followed the tutoring sessions, he asked me to explain why I tutored that way.

I told him simply that I have always hated having someone looking over my shoulder. Maybe it's just the personal space thing, but I can't function well that way. So, I just applied the Oriental concept of "Don't do to others what you don't want to have done to you." But there's another reason perhaps even as powerful for tutoring face to face across a table. You can see their facial expressions. And that very often is key to knowing whether or not they are comprehending a passage.

I started to explain why I wrote upside down as well as why I felt all experts in the field of teaching reading and writing should first teach themselves to read and write upside down and with their opposite hand before they promulgate their particular theory or theories about learning to read and to write. But I was stopped. Dr. Herman didn't think the members of the class needed to know my rationale.

I was getting close to having taken all the courses that Dr. Scruffy had felt I should take. Still I hadn't had a single committee meeting. Dr. Herman just followed Dr. Scruffy's lead. Since I had borrowed money and had to take at least twelve credit hours, Dr. Herman advised me to take some hours as dissertation hours, that is, paying for some of the 36 credit hours for the doctoral dissertation in advance. As it turned out, Dr. Herman got bit by a tick and got Lyme disease and was out for almost a year.

Although I tried to talk to him, I was told he didn't want to talk to me until he fully recovered and was back in school.

So, instead of getting a new committee chairperson, I began my research for my doctoral proposal. I began writing its rough draft. I wanted to make sure I would be able to get my Ph.D. degree on the same day in June, 1985 that my daughter Linda, her "twin" Steve, and my cousin's son Bob McCabe would be getting their B.S. degrees from Michigan State.

That was the wrong thing to do. When Dr. Herman returned to school and I informed him I had the rough draft of my thesis completed, he almost went beserk. He was furious. He insisted that I must first frame my research proposal and have it approved by the committee. Well, I had, but my committee had never met. He didn't care. He took one glance at my proposal and said it wasn't written properly. It was. It followed all the guidelines written. But it did venture into new territory, territory that Dr. Herman wasn't familiar with.

He said he wouldn't chair any doctoral candidate's committee if he didn't have the necessary expertise and knowledge to back the candidate's proposal. Only if I could find someone to work with me on my proposal and my thesis would he continue. He suggested the Linguistics Department. So I went there. And I did receive some backing. At least the head of the linguistics department did understand what I was trying to do. But since he wasn't part of the Education Department and my thesis had to do with a subject dealing with both linguistics and education, he refused to act as more than a part-time consultant for the thesis. Dr. Herman suggested that perhaps another expert from another college would be acceptable. I took him up on that. I knew that I could get Dr. Blue from the University of Iowa. Why? Because he and with the late Dr. Beemer had devised the *New Iowa Spelling Scale*. This was a major part of my statistical control for my thesis.

Then Dr. Herman just up and quit. Here I was. I had completed all my courses for my doctorate and had paid all my money for my thesis, but I had no chairperson for my committee. I went to the head of the education department. She made a few recommendations, and I contacted all those she recommended plus a few more. No one would accept the responsibility.

Then out of the blue, she called the first and the only meeting of my doctoral committee. Guess who chaired it? Dr. Herman, of course. The head of the education department and the assistant were there, to make sure I had a fair hearing. Uh, huh. Sure. And kangaroo courts are known for being outstandingly fair. Oh, one person was missing from my committee. Dr. Robert Trojanowicz, the Dean of the School of Criminal Justice. He was out of town. And he was familiar with the need for my doctoral research because it had to do with developing a quick valid measurement of reading ability for screening purposes in correctional facilities. Was it a coincidence that he was out of town? Bob was always someone I could trust. Hell, he was practically family to me. I knew him when he was in diapers. It took him a few more years to get to know me. And he knew and respected my work. Maybe I'm paranoid. But it doesn't mean that they weren't out to get me. And get me they did. The committee rejected my proposal for a thesis that had already been written. Two days later I received a letter from Michigan State University stating that I had been dropped from its doctoral program and was no longer eligible to take classes or to use any of its facilities.

Wow! I fired off a letter to the ombudsman's office. I had a string of very simple questions that could be answered yes or no, such as: Is it the policy of Michigan State University to not allow a second proposal to be given to a committee? Is it the policy of MSU for the head of a department to call the meeting instead of the doctoral student as it mandates in their rules and regulations? Is it the policy of MSU to allow the meeting to be conducted by the man who formally quit as both chairperson and as a committee member? The office of the ombudsman refused to answer a single question. They outright refused to do anything for me. I could drive all the way to

Lansing and discuss it with them, but they couldn't promise anything. No, I'm not paranoid. They were out to get me. But I remembered my grandfather's pet saying, "You can't win pissing battles with skunks."

But the time getting my ABT (All but thesis) instead of a Ph.D. wasn't a waste of time. I had learned a lot about what is wrong with schools of education. Yes, I suppose it's true that those who can, do. Maybe it's true that some of those who can't—become teachers. But I believe that there are just way too many "experts" who can't teach, who end up being responsible for teaching teachers how to teach.

Part III, Chapter 17

First things first. What needs to be taught?

WHENEVER I GIVE an inservice or workshop for teachers relating to reading, I am always challenged by some teacher or teachers who *only* want to discuss the best way to get students to comprehend what they're reading. To them reading is much more than just word calling. Reading has to be an interaction through print between the author and the reader. Wonderful, but first things first. My theory:

> Listening can be said to be a meaningful interaction between a speaker and a listener. If the sounds of speech are coming through a telephone line that has a bad connection, interaction cannot possibly take place. Understanding or comprehension depends upon hearing and interpreting correctly the sounds of speech.

My theory as it pertains to decoding in print:

> Listening can be said to be a ,rsmomhgi; omyrtsyopm between a spealrt smf s ;odyrmrt. If the dpimfd of speech are vp,omh through a telephone ;omr yjsy jsd a bad vpmmrvyopm, omyrtraction cannot [pddon;u take place. Imfrtdysmfomh or compreomdopm depends upon hearing omyrtxtryomh vpttrvy;u the sounds of speech.

First things first. *Let's fix the connection* so that all the sounds are heard properly. That's what decoding is all about. Making sure the student hears correctly in his head what the author intended that he hear.

If the telephone line is clear and the transmissions perfect and a person still doesn't understand, then it might be that the message contained words or phrases that are not within the recipient's vocabulary or experience. In which case, appropriate measures should be taken.

In school, there are occasional students who decode (or say the words perfectly) but who seemingly don't understand what they're reading. Many of these are the students who suffer from what I call the Pledge of Allegiance syndrome. For many students every single day starts with The Pledge of Allegiance. They recite it perfectly word for word. But ask them what it means to pledge allegiance, and they haven't the foggiest notion. All they know is

I pledge	We use this to dust with.
allegiance	a big important word
to the flag	stand facing the flag
of the United	opposite of U day'd
States	Texas, Utah, etc.
of America	part of USA
and to the republic	not a democrat
for which it stands	that's why we stand and and not sit during the pledge.
one nation	two less than three
under God	We pray to Her/Him/It
indivisible	You can't see us
with liberty	A bell with a crack in it.
and justice	the right to an attorney if you can't afford one.
for all	for us.

But it isn't the not knowing the meaning that constitutes what I call the Pledge of Allegiance Syndrome. It's the *not knowing* that they don't know.

Think about it. Many children (and adults) memorize prayers such as the Our Father and can recite them but woe unto the person who challenges them to explain any phrase of that prayer, especially "hallowed be Thy Name." It is the habit of just hearing pretty words with no meaning attached and *not knowing* that there is *no understanding* taking place. Yes, we laugh at children's misconceptions of phrases like Gladys the cross-eyed bear (Gladly thy cross I'd bear) or Harold be Thy name (Hallowed be Thy name).

To me it's simple.

The first step to improving reading comprehension is knowing what it is you don't know. Usually, it's what a word or a phrase means. In other words, vocabulary.

The second step to improving reading comprehension is developing a habit of thinking along with the reading.

Too many of us just hear a boring monotonous voice inside our skulls saying the words. That isn't interacting or reading. Some remedial teachers use various different materials designed to improve reading comprehension. The problem with most of them is that the students can't read all the words. And they guess. The object, of course, is to do the homework or classroom assignments and get a passing grade. Improving their reading isn't.

And how do I help students improve their reading comprehension? With humor! One of the many things I have my students do is to read short funny selections like the little anecdotes in *The Reader's Digest*.

Yes, I know it is the fashion of the intellectual snobs to look down on that magazine. But I like it, and I like to have a chuckle or two every day. And although I think it's good to have students enjoy reading, that's not the real reason for having them read short humorous selections. If they don't smile and chuckle once in a while, you know they're not comprehending. And because nobody likes to be the only one that doesn't get a joke, my students are more likely to check with me on the meaning of a phrase, and usually it's the key phrase that carries the pun.

I also use SRA's *Reading for Understanding* by Thelma Gwinn Thurston. But not quite the way the editors intended. I'm not interested in the "product" of a series of completed and self-corrected exercises. What good is doing a series of reading exercises in comprehension if you don't learn *why* you made the mistakes that you made? When they use the answer sheet to correct their paper, my students are expected to figure out why the kit's answer to a question is right and theirs is wrong. If they still think their answer is right, they're expected to make me teach them. Usually it has to do with a different meaning of a word they think they know, a word they didn't realize had more than one meaning.

Diagnosis and Testing

Frequently I receive phone calls from people who want someone tested for learning disabilities or for dyslexia. And I always ask them why. Why do they want the tests? If a test will help someone get the help they need, fine. But if they need help, why not just help them. Why bother with going through the rigamarole of testing? What are you going to accomplish besides making the student feel dumb?

I've always felt a little leery of places that both test specifically for learning disabilities and/or dyslexia and teach. To me it's too easy to make a case for conflict of interest. Besides, if someone comes to me for help, there's a reason. I don't need a test to determine that.

So when someone comes to me for help, I use the test that I wanted to use as the basis for my doctoral thesis. It's a first things first screening test. It's simple.

---

1. Can you write your name?

2. What day is today?

3. Can you read any of the following words?

   scrambled

   admitted

   accomplished

   misleading

   diseases

   humanity

If the answer to number 3 is no. The test is over. There's no need to embarrass him further. His knowledge of basic phonics is not in place.

If the answer to number 3 is yes, I ask him to read the words. If he correctly reads at least four of the words, I tell him that for the most part he has learned what he has been taught in school. Then I give him the second part of the test. But before I do, I tell him that this part covers words whose spelling contains phonic patterns that are not taught in any school. If he had any difficulty at all on the first part of the test, I can predict that he won't know any of the words on this part. If he breezed through the first part, I tell him he may only get one to three right on this part because this part of the test covers those words whose spelling contains phonic patterns that are not taught in any school.

---

4. Can you read any of the following words?

initialed

emphatic

fatigue

decoupage

attaché

entrepreneur

If the answer to that question is no. The test is over. No point in embarrassing the person anymore. If he says yes, then I ask him to read those words that he can. Very frequently it goes something like this:

in it tailed.
emp hatty ick
fat uh goo
de cup idge
attach
enter prenner

I always tell the person that they made good intelligent tries at the words. I tell them that the reason they missed them is not because they're dumb but because they haven't been taught these patterns.

I almost never give the rest of the survey tests. What's the point? I know what I have to do to help the person become a good reader.

First things, first. He has to be able to quickly and efficiently break the codes. Notice I said break the code**s**.

It was part of my thesis proposal that I would prove the existence of different codes within the English language of which only one is either systematically taught or encountered in the first three grades.

To humor Dr. George Herman I used academic names for the codes. But since I am no longer writing for him but for teachers and parents I use the following slightly more intelligible nomenclature:

English Spelling: The "Simple," the "Fancy," the "Insane," the "Tricky," and the "Scrunched up."[1]

My explanation is simplistic and not historically accurate. I know that. So please don't bother writing me and telling me what I already know. I use the following because it makes sense and is easier for a non-academic to remember even if it isn't quite true.

> A long time ago there was a place that had no name. It was filled with men and women who could do a lot of things. They could hunt deer. They could stand still and hide. They might kick a cat or pet the dog. They ran fast, played games and built houses. They might stop and start or jump up and down with joy. They had no bats to swing or balls to hit. Yet they did shout and scream and laugh and cry. To get food to eat they would spear fish and grow plants. They got milk from cows. They cut down trees to make houses. They grew grapes and made wine. At night they could watch the moon and stars. Or they could just go to sleep. Then came some more men in big boats from a place called Rome.

---

[1] The book with this title and the survey tests are available from the AVKO Educational Research Foundation.

Notice that the words in the box are all story-telling words. The base of all those words have but one syllable. Some can be expanded, for example, *hunt* can be expanded into *hunting* or *hunter* or *hunted*. But the base is still *hunt*. My story continues but this time in **bold** print are words that do not follow the normal phonic patterns of the story telling (actually tale-telling) language of the English people who first spoke the language we teach today in our schools during the first three grades.

This place is what today we call **England**. When the **Roman legions conquered** this island they **considered** the **indigenous** people **savages** who were **completely** without **culture** and **legal traditions**. **Naturally** they had to **educate** them. Since these **savages** had no **legal** terms or **cultural** terms in their **vocabulary**, the **Romans** added the **necessary** words from their **language** which was **Latin**. **Eventually** from **Ireland** and **Italy** came **missionaries** who brought **Christianity** to these **pagans**. These **missionaries** taught the **savages** that if they changed their **religion** from **polytheism**, were **baptized**, and **accepted Jesus** as their **savior**, **salvation** could be theirs. Because the **savages** did not have **appropriate** words in their **simple story** telling **language**, the **missionaries** added the words or **created** words from their two **favorite languages**, **Latin** and Greek. Then came the **Norman** French. They **conquered** the somewhat **civilized savages** added to their **vocabulary** words dealing with **cuisine** and **military matters**. So now words like **victuals**, **lieutenant**, **colonel, bivouac, rendezvous, boudoir**, and **unique** were added to the language. And as the **foreign** words **entered** the **language** they kept their **phonic patterns** rather than changing to the **phonic** spellings of the **original story**-telling **language** of the **savages**.

The readability of the two selections are:

	Simple Story-Telling	Fancy Educated
Flesch Kincaid	0.2	11.3
Coleman-Liau	2.8	14.4
Bormuth	7.1	10.9

As you can tell the words in bold print are additions to the original English story-telling language. These words also carry a great deal of meaning. It is impossible to teach any curriculum without using these big words. But you can tell tales without using big words. Or you can tell stories using just a few big words.

So what happens in the first three grades is that if phonics are taught students learn to read story-telling words like fish, ship, shop. shore, dish, wash, splash, etc., in which the /sh/ sound is always spelled /sh/. Even if they're not taught phonics but use the whole language or literature-based (story-telling) methods, they still learn that the letter combination sh is pronounced /sh/ because all the words that have that sound use those letters. The same is true with the vowel digraph -ou- which always has the same sound in little story-telling words like out, shout, scout, pound, sound, round, etc.

Now, dyslexics being of normal or above normal intelligence are also highly logical and desirous of being in control of the learning process. How then can they read a word like *precious*. "PREE see ouse" or "precky oh us" are just a few logical pronunciations given the phonics of the simple story-telling words. The sound /us/ is only spelled us or uss as in *bus*, *pus*, *thus*, *muss*, *fuss*, etc. The letter c has the sound of /k/ as in *cat* or /s/ as in *cent*. How then can a dyslexic come to the pronunciation "presh us" from *precious*?

One way is by sight methods which rely heavily on the shape and length of the word. Unfortunately the words *previous* and *precious* look a lot alike in the same manner as the number combinations 7839052 and 7836052 look a lot alike. Try teaching graduate students to read at least 220 words using a number code rather than letters. They will rebel. So would I. But even number codes can be simplified. For example this number-letter combination isn't very easy to remember with one glance. 8D01B0A2C13. But since this is the phone number (albeit scrambled) of the International Office of the Orton Dyslexia Society they make it easier to recall. Orton breaks it down into smaller components such as 1 (long distance) 800 (it's free) ABCD-123. There is no problem. 1-800-ABCD123. The longest component is the four digit ABCD. The others are one or three. Obviously 1-800-ABCD123 is easier to read and recall than 18002223123 or the scrambled 8D01B0A2C13.

Reading is first of all breaking the code. It's easier when you break the code into smaller units than the entire word.

Yes, I know that there are studies that say the opposite is true. But remember that these studies were all done on little children learning the story telling words of our language. Yes, sight methods will enable a six-year-old to respond quicker and more efficiently to a _small_number of words that are story-telling nouns faster than phonic methods. But let's look at a typical list of nouns that would be used for such a study:

1.	apple	14.	net
2.	bird	15.	owl
3.	cat	16.	pig
4.	dog	17.	queen
5.	elephant	18.	rat
6.	fire	19.	star
7.	girl	20.	table
8.	horse	21.	umbrella
9.	ice cream	22.	violin
10.	jar	23.	wall
11.	kite	24.	xylophone
12.	light	25.	yarn
13.	mother	26.	zebra

Notice that they are all nouns. They all can be used as key words to teach the alphabet. It is because of the method of word selection that a typical study is stacked in favor of sight methods.

Why? Because six-year-old students love to please their teacher. They can look at a card that has a picture of an elephant and say elephant. Their computer brain spots the fact that the word elephant is a big long word and it starts with an e. Automatic short cut time. Xylophone starts with an x and it's long. Short cut time. Children can be quickly taught to respond to xylophone but give them the word phone and they can't read it! And in a story the sentence, "The man got on an *ele*vator" is quite likely to come out as, "The man got on an *ele*phant!" But that is not part of the study.

It certainly takes much longer to teach all the phonic elements in those twenty five words. There are a minimum of 73 different patterns that would need to be taught.

But let's look at a different 26 words. Ready?

1.	rain	14.	straining
2.	rains	15.	stain
3.	rained	16.	stains
4.	raining	17.	stained
5.	train	18.	staining
6.	trains	19.	gain
7.	trained	20.	gains
8.	training	21.	gained
9.	trainer	22.	gaining
10.	trainers	23.	brain
11.	strain	24.	brains
12.	strains	25.	pain
13.	strained	26.	Spain

Let's count the patterns:

1. The -ain rime.
2. The r- onset

182

3. The -s suffix
4. The tr- onset
5. The -ed suffix
6. The str- onset
7. The -ing suffix
8. The st- onset
9. The -er suffix
10. The br- onset
11. The g- onset
12. The p- onset
13. The sp- onset

It is true that it will take longer to teach the 13 patterns necessary to decode the 26 -ain words than to teach the 26 nouns that contain 75 different patterns. But what a difference in transfer and utility and spelling!

But our leaders in the field of education don't bother doing studies on the "obvious" superiority of this method to teach beginning reading and spelling. Instead, they justify their approach to studies by invoking the sacred cow trinity of frequency, utility and grade level. Yes, grade level, schmade level.

On the next page is a simple chart of a few words by grade level: Remember grade levels are not determined by the intrinsic ease or difficulty in learning. Rather, the grade level of a specific word is determined by how frequently the word occurs in texts commonly used in grade schools and how often it appears in students' writings.

Grade 1	Grade 2	Grade 3	Grade 4	Grade 5 UP
funny ... fun				
away .... way				
nice		ice		
pink		ink		

table	able	
smile	mile	
still	till	ill
black	lack	
yellow	yell	low

As you can tell from the chart above that when words are taught by grade level, the word *nice* is taught in the first grade but *ice* isn't taught until the third. *Yellow* is a first grade word, but *yell* is third and *low* is fourth. Hmm. Strange. You would think the colleges would recognize that *ice* is in the active vocabularies of 1st graders and that they could use the word *ice* to teach the "rime" *ice* that is in words such as *nice, lice, slice, rice, price,* etc. But they don't. They also don't recognize that there is another -ice "rime" that rhymes with kiss and miss and **_not_** with **_ice_**. Notice that the word *notice* is not a compound word. It is not NOT-ICE. It doesn't rhyme with pot mice. Instead *notice* rhymes with "No kiss!" Compare the words that rhyme with ice and the words that rhyme with kiss.

ICE	KISS	KISS
ice	notice	bodice
lice	Alice	chalice
slice	office	Venice
nice	Janice	justice
rice	avarice	injustice
price	jaundice	lattice

ICE	KISS	KISS
spice	apprentice	pumice
splice	solstice	cowardice
mice	hospice	malice
dice	prejudice	Eunice
vice	practice	accomplice
advice	malpractice	dentifrice

For every additional -*ice* word that rhymes with *nice*, we can find two additional -*ice* words that rhyme with *kiss*, or even with *geese* as in *police*!

Author's interlude #3 Dr. Semmelweiss

Whenever I give an inservice or workshop I invariably have a teacher who dismisses the entire AVKO approach as simplistic. "The problem of illiteracy is a complex one. We should not be looking for simple solutions to complex problems."

Oh, that sounds so scientific. My answer to that has been the story of Dr. Semmelweiss. And it's been his story that has helped me maintain my sanity. But before I tell it, I ask my audience what scientific discovery has saved more lives than any other and who was responsible for it. "Penicillin!" is almost always shouted out with great enthusiasm and conviction. The audience is invariably amazed when I say, "Not even close." Then I give another clue. The discovery took place in 1842. Silence. Then I tell my story. Perhaps not as accurately as historians would prefer it, but since every accounting of his story I have read differs greatly in detail, I feel I have as much license to play the truth as the John Milton historians do. Anyway, here goes.

In 1842 in Vienna, Austria there was a university obstetrics hospital that had two separate wings. In one wing midwives were taught the art of delivering babies. In the other wing young medical students were taught the scientific method of delivering babies. The death rate just from puerpal (childbirth) fever was around 5% in the wing for training midwives, but was over 13% year after year in the wing for training doctors. The total death rate was over 50% because so many women died from hemorrhaging before they could contract the fever.

Now it came to pass that the head of the student wing went on a year's sabbatical. He appointed Semmelweiss to take his place. Now

Semmelweiss was a good Jewish boy who believed cleaniness was next to Godliness. So, as soon as his boss left he instituted some sweeping changes, like sweeping floors and even mopping them. He thought there ought to be clean sheets on the hospital beds for each new patient rather than having them changed once a month. He ordered the young medical students to wash and bleach out the stains in their smocks. The students objected. They acted just like high school football players who don't want to wear a perfectly clean uniform because that denotes no experience. So too, these young doctors-to-be felt that the more blood and pus stains on their smocks, the more their patients would respect them for their experience. But Semmelweiss wasn't having any part of that argument. Clean your smocks was the order of the day, every single day.

But Semmelweiss didn't stop there. He hated dirty hands and especially dirt underneath the fingernails. He ordered his students to wash their hands before they touched a patient. That was a strange order to the students. They hadn't heard about germs. Bacteria and viruses had not been discovered yet. And another quirk of Semmelweiss was that he couldn't stand the smell of the formaldehyde that was used to embalm the cadavers used by the students to practice Caesarian operations. Perhaps he was allergic to that chemical as are many people today. But allergies hadn't been invented yet. So what Semmelweiss did was to order his students to wash the smell off their instruments after each using in a chlorinated lime solution. That killed the smell and, of course, the germs that had been transmitted from the cadavers to the women. Now, the death rate from puerpal fever plummeted from over 13% down to less than 2% .

Semmelweiss instinctively knew that he was onto something. So when he attended medical conferences he tried to share with other doctors what he had learned. If you wash your hands and clean your instruments, women don't have to die from puerpal fever. Did the medical establishment listen to Semmelweiss? Does the educational establishment listen to McCabe? No. To admit that Semmelweiss was right would be to admit that they were butchering women by the thousands because they were too damn lazy to wash their hands. For today's educational establishment to admit that McCabe is right, they would have to admit that millions of Americans are needlessly illiterate because they refuse to teach phonics.

Back in 1842, Semmelweiss would not take no for an answer and kept screaming at doctors and surgeons to be clean. The medical establishment's answer was to have him committed to an insane asylum. I'm sure that there are many within the educational establishment today who would like to have McCabe locked up too for screaming out:

"Teach phonics! And do NOT limit the phonics taught to the phonics of the story-telling words. Make sure you teach the phonics of the the Latin, French, and Greek words that are used in everyday academic and recreational reading. In other words, teach the total phonics of the English language. And, while you're at it, let's teach the vocabulary of our English language and those phrases we have stolen from other languages. You know, those phrases our television writers and journalists just love to throw in, from the certain *je ne sais quois* of good-byes such as *ciao, sayonara, auf wiedersehen, shalom, salaam, aloha, dos svidanyah,* and *vaya con dios* to the obfuscatory legalese of *caveat emptor, modus operandi,* and *corpus delecti.* We shouldn't leave the teaching of these phrases to our foreign language teachers. For heaven's sake, how many languages can a student be expected to learn? Latin, Greek, French, Italian, Japanese, German, Hebrew, Russian and Spanish? Nonsense. Let's just include the most commonly used phrases as part of our reading vocabulary curriculum.

But I digress from my digression.

It might have amused Semmelweiss to know that although the concept of asepsis was ignored in his own country, his simple concept of Doctor-Wash-Your-Hands was spread to the United States by a Supreme Court justice and a poet—Dr. Oliver Wendell Holmes.

Sometimes I wonder who it will be that will spread my word that the phonics of our language must be taught intensively and systematically so that everybody can learn to read, so that words like _dyslexia_ and _dyslexics_ will become obsolete. I'm sure that it won't be me. I'm too old now for doing battle. Who will it be?

End of Author's interlude #3 Dr. Semmelweiss

Back to first things first. That there are distinctly different types of English words is not something that only McCabe has thought of. Marcia K. Henry, a distinguished educator and author of many books on the teaching of reading, a former president of the Disabled Reader Group of the International Reading Association (IRA) and currently (1994-95) president of the Orton Dyslexia Society writes about it. Her concept is more accademically acceptable than mine. She talks about English as having an Anglo-Saxon base with a layer of Latin followed by a layer of Greek.

Part III, Chapter 18

Breaking the code: Handwriting and Sequential Spelling.

BEFORE YOU CAN READ, you must have the tools to break the code of written language. In other words, you must know the alphabet and how it works. Not many experts will argue that point. But they will argue how much knowledge of the alphabet is necessary before children should be actively reading.

In one of the inservices that I gave not too long ago to a group of teachers in Iowa, I asked them to quickly demonstrate to me their knowledge of the alphabet by spelling the names of the letters. One after another they wrote: abcdefghijklmnopqrstuvwxyz or ABCDEFGHIJKL MNOPQRSTUVWXYZ.

When I told them that they were all wrong, they thought I was nuts. But they understood after I explained to them that there is a difference between a letter such as A and the many ways it can be written or printed and its many sounds ("ay" as in *ace*, "uh" as in *about*, "ah" as in *father*, "aw" as in *all*, and "a" as in *add*).

I then had them make a simple chart.

Letters	Sounds spelled in letters	Name spelled out in letters
Aa *Aa* **𝒶𝒶**	"AY," "ah," "uh" +	AY
Bb *Bb* **Bb**	"buh"	BEE
Cc *Cc* Cc	"kuh," "suh" +	SEE
Dd *Dd* Dd	"duh"	DEE
Ee *Ee* Ee	"EE," "e," +	EE
Ff *Ff* Ff	"fuh"	EFF
Gg *Gg* Gg	"guh" or "juh"	JEE
Hh *Hh* Hh	"huh"	AY'ch
Ii *Ii* Ii	"ah'ee" or "i" +	AH'ee
Jj *Jj* Jj	"juh"	JAY
Kk *Kk* Kk	"kuh"	KAY
Ll *Ll* Ll	"luh" or "ul"	EL
Mm *Mm* Mm	"muh"	EM
Nn *Nn* Nn	"nuh"	EN
Oo *Oo* Oo	"OH" or "AH" +	OH
Pp *Pp* Pp	"puh"	PEE
Qq *Qq* Qq	"kuh"	K'yoo
Rr *Rr* Rr	"ruh" or "ur"	AR (or AH'r)
Ss *Ss* Ss	"suh"	ESS
Tt *Tt* Tt	"tuh"	TEE
Uu *Uu* Uu	"OO" or "uh" +	YOO
Vv *Vv* Vv	"vuh"	VEE
Ww *Ww* Ww	"wuh"	DUB'L Yoo
Xx *Xx* Xx	"zuh" or "ks"	EKS
Yy *Yy* YY	"yuh"	WAH'ee
Zz *Zz* Zz	"zuh"	ZEE

Did the teachers all agree with the way I spelled the sounds and the letters? Of course not. I don't agree with myself on some of them. But they all agreed on the one essential point: that is, the names, sounds, and spellings of letters are different one from the other. Now, they understood why the names and the sounds of the letters can easily become confused in a student's mind.

The teachers also were able to see that naming the letters of the alphabet is a rather formidable task because there are far more than 26 configurations to learn. For example, the letter A has a minimum of 6 different common configurations: A, a, A, ɑ, *ɑ*, *a*. If we eliminate teaching the cursive letters *ɑ*, *a* we still have over 70 different configurations to learn to name using only 26 names.

But naming the letters is only one task. Learning alphabetic order is another. Learning the sounds that letters make (or don't make) is even more formidable.

So how do schools generally approach this task? They teach the names of *all* the letters first. And that sounds like a logical approach. Certainly, it's the traditional approach. But is it the right approach? I don't think so.

First of all, when a child comes to school, what does he expect and want to do? He wants to learn to read and write—not name letters! So rather than capitalize on their initial enthusiasm, we teach just about everything children need to know except reading and writing in kindergarten. For one whole year the students are kept waiting. Developmentalists will say most kindergarteners are not ready for reading and writing. But how can that be? They have already learned to speak and understand the basic spoken language of English. Not perfectly, of course, but if they come from an English speaking home, they do know the basic words and are learning new words at a fantastic rate.

And this is without having a class in English taught by a certified English teacher or speech therapist! They learned by themselves. First, they learned the body language of touch; then, the tone of language. Did you ever notice how everybody automatically slips into a different higher pitched tone when they talk to a baby? Babies learn to respond first to tones of love and alarm. And they begin to learn how to manipulate the adults around them with their coos and their cries. And somehow they begin to crack the code.

Now when I'm going through an explanation of this, I suddenly shift into the Russian language and begin what sounds like a whole lot of jibberish to the audience. Actually it's merely a poem that I memorized while I was learning Russian at the Army Language School. I remind my audience in English, of course, of how difficult it is to reproduce a sound that you hear. And I give them the word **БЫЛЬ** (Russian for "was"). It contains a vowel sound that does not exist in English. They try and fail. They try and they fail. And of course so do babies. But babies don't give up trying. Eventually they learn to reproduce correctly most of the sounds. True, I didn't. As you know, I had to have four years of rather intensive speech therapy at Cook School.

The point is—a child who enters kindergarten has already accomplished the most difficult linguistic feat of all, learning to speak a language, learning to decode and encode the spoken word. Compared to that, learning to decode and encode the written word is a piece of cake or rather, should be a piece of cake.

Personally, I don't think a child would ever learn to speak if he first had to master the naming jargon of speech before he employed it. Children don't have to learn terms such as voiced and unvoiced, glottal stops and bilabial fricatives before they learn to speak.

Likewise, they really don't have to learn all the names of the letters of the alphabet before they start learning to read. We can teach the letter A. We can tell the students its name is "AY" and it has a number of different sounds. When it's all by itself it's a real word and its sound is "uh." I prefer to make sure that the students know that it doesn't matter whether the letter A is written **A, a, A,** *a,* or even *a,* *a,* its last name is the same but its first name is Capital (or BIG) or Small as the case may be. But all by itself the letter is a word. And we practice writing the manuscript *A.* Certainly I would prefer kindergarten teachers to employ the multi-sensory methods of teaching the writing of the letter as preached by the followers of the

Slingerland or Orton Gillingham approaches. But I can't blame them. Their college professors in the colleges of education across the country do not and probably will not teach these multi-sensory techniques unless they are forced to.

Anyway, after A comes B. And guess what? We have a word! BAA as in BAA BAA BLACK SHEEP. Right off the bat the children are forced to learn that the letter A has more than one sound. And I believe we should teach the children that *B* has the name Capital BEE and *b* has the name Small Bee and the sound "buh."[1]

With the letter C comes A CAB. And also a third sound for the letter A. With D comes DAD and BAD. And as long as the stick-ball method of teaching letter formation is NOT used, there is very little danger of students confusing the *b* and the *d*. With E comes ED and ED in BED. Also we have BE and BEE. With F comes FEED and FED.

My personal order of presentation pretty much follows the alphabet. I teach ABCD one letter at a time. I also teach my students the first principles of alphabetic order. Then I stick in RST. I teach *them* one letter at a time. As I need the *r* for *br cr* and *dr* blends, I may spend many days locking in the letter *r* and its blends with *b*, *c*, and *d* as well as reviewing ABCD. I need the *s* for plurals and the *t* for the very important -*at* family and the *TR* blend. After teaching the RST, I then return to alphabetic order with EFGHIJK. Each is taught separately to mastery. At this point my students can recite abcdefghijk and can tell what letter comes before and after any letter. They can put words using these letters in alphabetical order.

Then I stick in Y so I can change words such as *trick* and *dad* into *tricky* and *daddy*. And while they are mastering the stroke that makes the letter *y*, they are also learning words such as *try*, *dry*, *cry*, and *fry*

---

[1] "I have no quarrel with those who do not want to add the schwa sound "uh" to an initial consonant. In fact, in my personal teaching I define consonants as shapers and vowels as grunts. I don't believe that there is only one way of teaching phonemic awareness.

and how the *y* changes into an *i* in *tries, dries, cries, fries, tried, dried, cried,* and *fried.*

Then LMNOPQ. Each letter is taught separately and the patterns it comes in. For example, with *l* comes the initial sound, the *l* blends with *b* (blend), *c* (click), *f* (flick) and has the *all, ell, ill* family sounds as well as the *al, ale, ail, eel, eal, ile, alt,* and *alk* families.

When I get to *Q* I just have to teach *U.* Since we had RST and Y very early on we now have ABCDEFGHIJKL MNOPQRSTU and continue on with VWX and Z.

By the time my students have finished learning the alphabet they can do much more than just recite the names of the letters. They can use the alphabet. They can read correctly any regular one syllable word and correctly spell most of them. In fact, they can usually read and spell new one syllable words correctly the first time they encounter them.

For more information on the handwriting system I have developed for teaching reading and spelling, see *AVKO Sequential Handwriting* in the Appendix under the heading of AVKO Materials.

Sequential Spelling

One of my friends once said to me, "McCabe, just as it might take a thief to catch a thief, it just might take a dyslexic to teach a dyslexic. But it takes more than just a dyslexic, it takes a total non-comformist to come up with your way (Sequential Spelling) to teach spelling."

I suppose I have to plead guilty to some degree of non-conformity. After all, most spelling programs require that students study a list of words. But I don't believe in studying. I believe in learning. Note: Studying and learning are two different things. I have always contended that the things we know best, the things we learned best, we did **not** study. For example, I never studied the names of my relatives. And it seems I've always known them. But do I know the names of all the states and all the provinces in Canada, their capitals, their two largest cities, their rivers, as well as their agricultural and/or industrial products? Not now I don't. But when I was in the 5th grade at Cook School I thought I knew them. I scored 100% on the test. I had memorized all those facts. My 100% on that test which simply measured recall only meant that my short term memory was working, and that my sister Betty June knew how to tutor me for tests. It did not accurately measure my permanent knowledge of American/Canadian geography.

And of course there is that little matter of equity. On a standard pretest of twenty words, the A student will miss no more than two. The B student will miss no more than five. The C student will miss at least five but no more than ten. But the D/E student and the dyslexic student will miss at least fifteen. In other words, in order to score a perfect 100% on Friday, the A student only has to learn two words at most, the B student only has to learn five words at most, but the D/E or dyslexic student has to learn at least fifteen words. He can learn five times as many words as the A student and still fail the test on Friday. Something is wrong here.

And what is wrong is what the poor student learns. He learns that he is dumb. No matter how hard he studies he still flunks. He has to be dumb. That's what he thinks. Now the C student who only had to learn five to ten words, learns just enough of them (like 20%) to get at least a C on the test. By Monday he has forgotten what he had learned. But what the heck, it doesn't matter. He has learned that the only thing that's important is the grade on the test. He knows that the grade won't change even if he forgets how to spell all the words.

Yes, I plead a bit of non-conformity here. I don't think students should be learning that what's important is the grade on a spelling test. I think they should be learning to spell.

So I eliminate the study. But I don't eliminate the testing—just the red pencil and the grading. What I hit upon was a natural outgrowth of my word family approach to decoding. Remember how I would help a student learn to decode (read) the word advice? I would have him write the word ice in green about ten times. Then I would have him spell different words that rhymed with *ice* and write the beginning letters in red.

ice
dice
nice
lice
slice
rice
price
mice
vice
advice

For me, it was just a natural logical progression to adapt this concept to teaching spelling. What I would do is to give the word **ice**. The students would attempt the spelling. Then I would give the correct spelling. And then each student would correct his own spelling. None of this pass-your-paper-to-the-person-behind-you bit. I still remember that little girl behind me giggling and then telling the whole class that I had left out the **r** in **shirt**. Only the way she said it wasn't quite that kind.

Years later when I did a review of the literature on spelling for my doctoral thesis, I discovered that about the only thing that moderately successful spelling programs had in common was student self-correction.[1] But that shouldn't have been a surprise. Programmed learning and teaching machines and computer-assisted instruction use that very principle. But it is the careful sequencing of the words that makes the student self-correction work so well. In many ways, it's like teaching a child to catch a ball. You don't hand him a baseball glove and ask Nolan Ryan to throw his fast ball to him. You start up

---

[1]"The child correcting his own spelling test, under the direction of the teacher, is the single most important factor in learning to spell." See Robert J. Fitzsimmons and Bradley M. Loomer, *Spelling: Learning and Instruction.* Iowa City, IA: Iowa State Department of Public Instruction and The University of Iowa, 1978., p. 30.

close and throw easy. As he approaches mastery of the simple catch, you move back just a little and continue throwing the ball to him. Bit by bit and day by day you increase the distance and the speed until catching a ball is automatic.

So too I start with the slow pitch. My students learn from their mistakes rather than being punished by red check marks splashed like blood all over their papers. And I noticed two very significant changes in my students, both of which are essential to self-esteem. One, they weren't as upset at missing a word on my tests because, after all, they hadn't studied the word. Two, quite often they correctly spelled a word that they had never seen nor heard nor spelled before. Dumb people can't do that. Only somebody with intelligence can spell a word right without ever having seen it before!

Unfortunately, not all teachers understand the concept of immediate student self-correction. When I was teaching at Zimmerman Junior High a special education teacher complained to me about one of her students who just couldn't spell. I offered her a copy of my newly developed *Sequential Spelling* and carefully explained to her how to use it. Or at least I thought I had carefully explained it to her. About two weeks later she saw me in the teachers' lounge and told me that my *Sequential Spelling* didn't work. That puzzled me. It had always worked before! So I asked her how she was doing it. She told me she gave the girl the test and then handed the book to her to correct her paper.

Of course, she was getting them all wrong. I again explained to the teacher, that the student got the opportunity to correct her mistake after each and every word—not after the whole test was over. "Oh," was all she said. I advised her to start all over again with lesson 1. She did. And surprise! This time the *Sequential Spelling* worked for her student.

There's another little hitch in giving these tests that can prevent learning from taking place. Some students so hate to make mistakes that they won't attempt to spell the word until after the correct spelling is given. No matter how often I warn teachers about this, there are always a few who just sit behind their desk and don't watch over all their students. Those teachers who walk around the room and monitor their students get the best results.

Part III, Chapter 19

Some Parents Need Help to Help Tutor Their Kids. Where are our schools when we need them?

DYSLEXICS ARE SOMETIMES ACCUSED of being slow learners. There's no doubt in my mind that in some areas I'm very, very slow to learn. For example, even though I had to teach my own dyslexic son to read, it never dawned on me that there are other parents who have kids having problems in school who want to know how to help their kids.

It just never occurred to me. At least not until a parent who just happened to be a member of the Flint Board of Education, Leo Soda, came to the foundation to talk to me about helping his son. He told me that like a good parent he went to all his son's parent-teacher conferences. He knew his son was having problems learning. The teachers, one after another, said that he would catch up. It's just a matter of time. So they passed him and passed him and passed him all the way up to the 7th grade—and still he hadn't learned to read and write above a third grade level.

I demonstrated to Mr. Soda that his son wasn't dumb by running through my Sequential Spelling routine. I had his son attempt the spelling of "scattered" as in the sentence, "You shouldn't have scattered your tools all over the place." He didn't want to write anything. So I asked him to just put down whatever letters he thinks might be in the word. So, he put down **s-d-a-r.** I congratulated him. I told him even though he didn't spell the word **scattered**, every letter he put down was in that word. Then I told him that the next time I asked him to spell the word **scattered** he would spell it 100% correctly.

"No way, man. No way!" was his reply. But you know, by the time I walked him through it. He did. The first word I had him attempt to spell was *at*. He snickered. But he spelled *et*. I wrote the word *at* and asked him to erase the *e* and make it an *a*. Then I gave him *bat*. This time he spelled *bat* correctly even though he had misspelled *at*. I congratulated him. Then I gave him *rat*. He spelled *rat* correctly. And I congratulated him. Then I gave him *brat*. He wrote *bat* hesitantly. He knew *brat* needed some other letter but he didn't know what. I told him that I teach backwards. And I wrote *at* and told him he got the important sound right. I told him he got the first sound right. But somehow he didn't quite hear the *rat* (and then I added the *r* to the *at*) in *brat*. Then I added the *b* to the *rat* to make *brat*.

Aha! I could see the light turn on.

This is Lesson 1 that I gave:

at
bat
rat
brat

Then I had Leo Soda's son turn over his paper, and for about ten minutes I talked about the nature of memory. I went into my normal spiel about how psychologists have oversimplified the concept of memory into just two categories, short term and long term. In reality there are many types. The following examples pertain to me. Some lucky people can remember another person's name for years and years with only one introduction—but not me.

Length of memory	*Personal examples of things I can sometimes remember for that duration.*
Split second	Sense data such as visual images of cars, trees, fire hydrants, billboards, etc., images and sounds I hear while I'm driving a car.
Seconds	Processed verbal data such as words and sentences. It only took me a few seconds to type from the top of this page to here. The number of sentences you can recite word for word is about the length of this type of short term memory. Mine is horrible.
Minutes	Processed concepts such as names of people I have been introduced to. Many times I forget names within seconds instead of minutes.
Hours	An interesting hand at the bridge table, the bidding, and the play. Most I forget within minutes.
Days	What the weather was like and what I had for dinner or some historical facts presented in a class. A really exciting bridge hand.
Weeks	Something I was asked to do and didn't.
Months	Names of people that I have made a conscious effort to learn and to use every day. If I stop seeing them and stop using their names, I forget them.

Years	Names of people that are important to me. These people are people that I see regularly. If I stop seeing them for years, I am liable to forget their names. A bidding sequence or incident at a bridge tournament which had special significance to me. Usually it was a mistake I shouldn't have made.
Decades	Names of people (maybe) that are very important to me or the sounds of their voices. Even if I don't see them for ten or fifteen years, I still remember them, name or voice but not necessarily both. For example, while I was at Gordon and Sue Parnes' house, the phone rang. Sue left the room to answer it. A minute later she called to me and asked me to come to the phone. "Do you know who this is?" was what I heard.
	"Of course," I said. "How can I forget your attempt to play Scott Jopin's *The Entertainer* between sessions at the Midland Bridge Tournament?"
	I had instantly recognized Gordon's former steady bridge partner Dan Suty's voice but I didn't recall his name.
Lifetime	The English language. Names of my brothers and sisters and close relatives (except when I have to make introductions). My birthday. Hopefully, my wife's birthday and our anniversary. How to ride a bike.

I then pointed out to the board member Leo Soda and his son David that it was important to let some time pass so that he had time to forget. Then I went to the second lesson.

bats
rats
brats
flat
flatter
spat

David spelled **bas** for **bats**. I congratulated him on his good hearing. Leo looked puzzled. But then he leaned back and nodded affirmatively as I explained.

"There are only three phonemes in **bats**. **B**uh **a**aaa and ₜ**S**ssss.[1] To say **B**uh **a**aa **t**uh ₜ**S**ssss you would have to spit. Just try to say **bat** and then ₜ**S**ssss. You can't say it without spitting. But we just have to spell **bat** and then add the **s**.

David got **rats** right. He almost missed **brats**, but then he remembered the **rat** in **brat** and spelled it correctly. He left out the **l** in **flat**. But I congratulated him for getting the first letter right and the last two. I wrote **lat** and said **lat** and then I added the **f** and said **fffff- lat**. He corrected his error. Then I gave **flatter**. David spelled it **flatr**. Again I congratulated him. He got the **flat** part right. And I told him that he got the **r** sound right, except that in our language we like to use a lot of letters. We just have to double the **t** and add **er** just to get the **atter** sound. He spelled **sat** for **spat**. Again I congratulated him for hearing the correct beginning and ending sounds. I wrote **at**, added the **p** making it **pat** and then put the **s** in front of **pat** and said **sss-pat**.

---

[1]In Russian they have a special letter for this phoneme: Ц

I then went into my explanation that the natural way of learning was by making and correcting our own mistakes. This is the way we learn to stand up, to walk, to talk, and to use a knife and fork and drink out of a glass. Since he had a little sister, David could understand that indeed while he was learning to feed himself he too had got his baby food up his nose and in his ears and all over the floor.

Then I went into the third lesson.

Lesson 1 Lesson 2 Lesson 3

Lesson 1	*Lesson 2*	*Lesson 3*
bat	*bats*	*batted*
rat	*rats*	*ratted*
brat	*brat*	*batter*
	flat	*flats*
	flatter	*flatters*
	spat	*spats*
		mat
		matter
		hat

David spelled **badid** for **batted**. "That's a great misspelling!" I told him. "That's exactly how it sounds. However, we first spell the word **bat**, double the **t** and add **ed**. David corrected his error.

When I gave **ratted**, he was ready for it. I could almost read his lips as he said silently to himself, **rat, double** the **t** and add **ed**. He spelled **battr** for **batter** and felt a little embarrassed that he had forgotten the **e**. But I congratulated him for getting the **bat** and doubling the **t** and getting the **r** sound. He spelled **fats** for **flats** but before I could correct him, David corrected himself. Leo Soda smiled and nodded. He could see what I was doing and why it was working. Best of all, he could see that David wasn't dumb. The rest of the words on lesson three David got right.

We talked for a few minutes. Leo Soda wanted to know why his son didn't learn like the other kids in his class from the regular spelling books. He knew that according to the nonverbal IQ tests his son had been given that his son wasn't dumb, not by a long shot. His son had an IQ of 121. Why couldn't he learn? I could have gone into a long spiel about learning styles, learning differences, specific learning disabilities, and dyslexia, but I didn't. Instead, I told Leo that his son David had a very logical mind. The problem was that when he tried to apply what he had been taught about spelling and phonics, nothing seemed to work. I showed David the word **precious**. He tried to read it and it came out "preeky ouse." After telling David that he had been taught that *c* has only two sounds (/k/ or /c/), I explained that there is no logical way he could be expected to know that the letters *ci* in **precious** and words like **special** and **suspicion** are pronounced /sh/. He had been taught that the letters **ou** make the /ou/ sound as in **out**, **pout**, **shout**, etc. How can you logically get the sound "**us**" from "**ous**"?

Then I went on to Lesson 4.

Lesson 1	Lesson 2	Lesson 3	Lesson 4
bat	bats	batted	batting
rat	rats	ratted	ratting
brat	brat	batter	batters
	flat	flats	pat
	flatter	flatters	flattered
	spat	spats	spatter
		mat	mats
		matter	matters
		hat	hats
			cat
			scat
			scatter

David had a little problem with **flattered**. So I walked him through it with, "Spell **flat**, change **flat** to **flatter** and then add your **ed** to get **flattered**." I explained to his father that knowing sounds are not enough. I told him I could spell the "urd" sound 14 different ways as in b**ird**, st**irred**, w**ord**, lab**ored**, lab**oured**, stand**ard**, coll**ared**, c**urd**, occ**urred**, pict**ured**, h**erd**, h**eard**, def**erred**, ent**ered**, euch**red**.

When I got down to the word **cat**, David heaved a big sigh as if to say, "Why cat? Everybody can spell **cat**." When I gave **scat**, I could almost see his mind churning away. He had started to write **sk** and then changed his mind and wrote **scat** with a decisive flourish. When I asked him to spell **scatter**, he whipped right through it. He knew he was going to get it right. And of course he did spell **scatter** correctly. Then I showed him how he had spelled it about twenty minutes earlier: **sadr**.

Leo Soda was now convinced of two things. One, his son wasn't dumb and could learn. Two, he wasn't ever going to learn in the special education classes or regular classes in the Flint Public Schools. He would have liked to have his son take advantage of AVKO's free daily tutoring, but his time was too valuable. He just couldn't afford to bring him out every day. He asked if I could work with him once a week. My answer was no. I knew that he could afford to pay me $100.00 an hour, but I told him that tutoring once a week would be a waste of my time, David's time, and his money. To get the patterns of English spelling locked into David's computer brain, David would have to use them every day. His computer brain must be convinced of the necessity of putting the patterns into the permanent instantly retrievable memory bank.

I offered to teach Leo or his wife how to work with David or to teach someone of their choosing who could tutor his son on a daily basis. But Leo ended up doing something else. Now that he knew his son could learn to read and write, Leo took him out of the Flint Public Schools and sent him to a private school in North Carolina that specializes in working with learning disabled youngsters.

Leo Soda could do that because he was rich. But what about the rest of us just plain folks? How many of us could send our kids away to a private school like that? That got me thinking. Why can't we teach parents to tutor their kids?

The logical place for teaching parents how to tutor would be in the adult community education programs. So because I don't believe in re-inventing wheels I first tried to discover whether or not any such classes were offered anywhere. At that time the AVKO Foundation was sending a newsletter to every school system in Michigan as well as to its members all across the country. We offered a $100.00 reward for information concerning any school system that offered a class for parents in how to tutor their youngsters.

We had two educators apply for the the $100.00 reward. One was a from an adult community education director from Coldsprings who showed as evidence a brochure that listed a course offering for parents entitled "Helping Your Child Learn to Read." When I asked to talk to the teacher about the course, he answered rather sheepily, "We couldn't find a teacher for it. But we did offer the course and parents did sign up for it. Doesn't that count?"

It might have. But I did find one small school system in Northern Michigan that actually had a class for parents. It wasn't exactly what I had in mind. But it was a good idea. It was for parents who wanted to help their kids in kindergarten and first grade. They were learning what it was that the school was teaching to their youngsters so that they could assist them at home. Not a bad idea. More schools should do the same. And maybe they are with Chapter 1, Title 1 funds. So AVKO gave them the $100.00.

But armed with the knowledge that there were no adult community education programs for parents who want to help their children overcome reading/spelling problems, I decided to develop a course. I began writing lesson plans. Then I contacted the Clio Area Schools. I talked to the Community School Director Richard Nottingham, and he seemed rather enthusiastic. I told him that as a new class it would have to be really advertised. He agreed and said that he would take care of it. His idea of really advertising was to just include it right in the middle of all the other classes for cake decorating and dog obedience. But somehow or another I ended up with about ten parents.

At the end of the first session, a Mrs. Schott came up and showed me a spelling test that her daughter had taken. Mrs. Schott said her daughter Laura was a nervous wreck. Then she pointed out to me the teacher's notation that Laura had not written her words seven times each. "That's not true," Mrs. Schott said, "Laura *drew* each word exactly seven times." I was amazed at Mrs. Schott's choice of the word *drew* rather than *wrote*. It showed me that she really understood a great deal about Laura's problem.

I started to demonstrate to her how she could use the Sequential Spelling technique with her daughter. "I really don't have the time to do all that," Mrs. Schott said to me. "Don't you have something already put together that I can use?"

I did. I had my Sequential Spelling I-V. I showed her how to use it. I also asked her to please not help her daughter with her regular school spelling words. This rather surprised her. But when I explained to her that what is important for Laura to learn is spelling—not grades on spelling tests, she began to understand. And she did tell Laura, as I asked her to, that she didn't care at all about grades on spelling tests. Nobody has ever asked me what grade I got on any spelling test in any grade. How about you? How many times have you been asked what grade you got on the spelling test you took on the second Friday in November when you were in the fourth grade?

The class I taught lasted seven weeks. And we covered all kinds of different issues, including but not limited to motivation, comprehension, and reading speed. On the last night of class Mrs. Schott showed me the last three tests in spelling that Laura had. They were all perfect papers. See p. 209 to see what her first perfect 100% paper looked like:

Laura Schott's first paper before her mother took my class in tutoring..

Note the absence of any positive comments on Laura's perfect paper. Both teachers and parents are human. We all tend to be generous with criticism and stingy with praise. I believe we should all try to reverse that and be generous with praise and stingy with criticism. Those who took the class seemed to enjoy it. They all said that they got a lot out of it and that their children's reading had really started to improve. When the course ended I gave all the evaluations to the community school director. He seemed pleased. But he never found a teacher to replace me even though I told him I would help the teacher through it and provide all the materials free.

I ended up teaching that same course in two other nearby small towns. And with the same results. They would have a class if I would teach it. They wouldn't try to recruit a teacher within their system to do it.

But it wasn't a loss. I learned several important things: Even parents who claim they don't have the patience to work with their children *can learn* to have patience. The first night of class is when the parents have the greatest amount of enthusiasm and the least amount of expertise. Parents want something to get results with NOW! So what did I do? I wrote a special version of my Sequential Spelling for parents and a special response book for their children. But because some of the children might be teenagers, I made sure that the sentences were not putdowns. I've always felt that you can treat a child as an adult, but you should never treat an adult as a child. No matter how good your lesson plans are, you won't be able to follow them. But if you don't have lesson plans, you'll find that you need them.

Then I re-wrote my own lesson plans and made sure that during the first class meeting the parents would be taught how to use the books at home. That way on the second meeting of the class success stories could be told.

The last thing that I did was to write a pamphlet on how to go about setting up a class for parents who want to learn how to tutor. These AVKO gives away free.

> We would like to give copies of this pamphlet to every PTA, to every Chapter 1, Title 1 Parent Group, and to every board of education member, and every principal in the country.

Unfortunately, AVKO doesn't have that much money. And at this writing, there hasn't been a single charitable foundation interested in funding such a project. If you happen to know of one, please ask them to contact us. The reason is simple. Everytime someone tells us we really ought to contact this foundation or that foundation, we are told by the same foundations that although they believe it is a most worthy cause, it doesn't quite fit in with their pattern of giving.

We believe that there is not a single charitable foundation whose pattern of giving would include giving money to help spread the concept that when students encounter learning-to-read or learning-to-spell problems in school and require daily one-to-one tutoring, schools can best help them by training their parents (or friends or other relatives) to be volunteer tutors.

Boy, would we love to have you prove that we're wrong.

Part III, Chapter 20

The AVKO
Word Difficulty Dictionary

IN DOING MY RESEARCH for my doctoral thesis, I ran across Harry Greene and Brad Loomer's *The New Iowa Spelling Scale*. It was (and is) a fascinating study. What they did was to make a spelling list of 5,517 of the most commonly used words in students' writings. Naturally, in the making of this list, they consulted all the major word lists of their day and used them to justify the inclusion or exclusion of specific words. For example, proper names such as Jesus and Buddha were excluded. Then after they compiled the list they enlisted the aid of schools all across the country to test their students on these words. Then afterwards they analyzed the data they had collected.

The New Iowa Spelling Scale						
Grade 2	3	4	5	6	7	8
babies 2	11	21	49	70	78	88
baby 44	74	76	90	92	95	97
back 39	57	85	93	98	99	99
.....						
bankruptcy ...	2	3	3	9	17	19
banquet 1	2	6	14	34	56	69

Each number represents the percentage of students in the grade that can correctly spell the word during the month of September of that grade.

One of the first things that I noticed was that the words were listed in alphabetical order. Yes, it didn't take a stroke of genius to notice that. But I have always been interested in teaching easier words first. On the five listed above it's easy to see that the word *back* is the easiest and *bankruptcy* is the most difficult. And it's not hard to do the ranking of *back, baby, babies, banquet* and *bankruptcy* in order of ease of learning. But it's not so easy with over 5,000 words to do that.

At that time we had a CPT word processor that could do simple math. So, I re-entered almost all the data. Talk about boring repetitive work! But I did it. AVKO didn't have the money to hire someone to do it for us. The data I did not include was the data on the 2nd through fourth grades because so many of the 5,000 words were not given to these early elementary students. So because all the words were given only to the fifth through eighth grades, I just entered the data on those grades. I then averaged them. That gave me the percentage of 5-8th graders that could spell a given word. I then used the word processor's capability of alphabetizing by numbers and put them in that order.

But there was something about the percentages that I didn't like. First of all, every school is different. Just because 99% of the students in one school might be able to spell the word *back* doesn't mean that you should expect all schools to achieve that percentage. Likewise, just because the national average was 71.25% for spelling the word *babies*, I don't believe a school should be satisfied with being above average with a 75% score. To me, I wouldn't be satisfied with anything less than 98% for that word.

So what I did was to rank order the words by using a scale of 1-21 with 1 representing the very easiest word—one which everyone can spell and 21 a word so difficult that no one can spell it. Using a simple formula I translated the averages. And so I now was able to have two separate arrangements of the words. One was by order of difficulty in which the words were listed.

1.00	I, a	
1.05	in is	
1.10	you he out	
1.15	good it me old one see she ten up	
1.20-19.35	...(I only left out about 5,000 words here)	
19.40	criticism accommodation lieutenant affidavit	
19.80	efficiency indefinitely	
20.10	psychology	

The other way was alphabetical but with a twist. Now I included all the words that had the same level of difficulty right next to it.

babies	6.75	coach cheering refund blessing
baby	2.30	noon note who any called
back	1.55	if add away call room cat new
bankruptcy	18.60	conscience endeavor
banquet	12.35	policy affection justified rarely

This now enabled me to devise a method to test the effectiveness of any school's spelling program. I could give a spelling test with half the words being those that were in their spelling program. The other half would be words of equal difficulty but were not in their spelling program. If the spelling program were to be really effective there would be a significant difference[1] between the pairs of word equivalents.

---

[1]By significant I do NOT mean statistically significant. Educational studies ɛ filled with statistically significant findings that have no real practical application.

For example, if the words *babies, baby, back, bankruptcy* and *banquet* were all to be in a school's spelling list somewhere before the fifth grade, you could have them as the odd numbered words. You could then use the even numbers to put words of equivalent difficulty that were not in their spelling list. The following could be such a ten word test.

1.	babies	2.	coach
3.	baby	4.	note
5.	back	6.	room
7.	bankruptcy	8.	conscience
9.	banquet	10.	affection

The number of students who correctly spelled *coach* would represent the number of students who would have correctly spelled babies without having studied it! Thus the difference between the number who got babies right and coach right would represent the number who really learned from the spelling series. What I have found out and most teachers have suspected for years is that the spelling books used in our school systems just don't help the students learn to spell. So if out of 150 students the results show that there were ten more correct spellings on the odd numbered words than the even, it could mean that ten students actually learned one word each that they wouldn't have learned just from doing their daily school work and their own reading and writing for pleasure. But the statisticians would say that it showed a significant statistical difference. Big deal. Yes, sarcasm is intended.

Part III, Chapter 21

Get outta my face!
Get offa my case!

IN MANY THINGS, I'm an awfully slow learner. It took me almost twenty years after "discovering" that words have spelling patterns, that phrases and sentences have patterns, too.

No, I'm not referring to the traditional grammatical patterns described by the terms nouns, verbs, adjectives, adverbs, prepositions, conjunctions, simple, compound and complex. What I'm referring to has to do with the inner language of emotion and action that is connected to the words we choose to use. In other words, the hidden psychology of speech.

As I recall, I first really formulated this concept when I was on the 19th hole at the Clio Golf Club. Our foursome had somehow got diverted from telling golf stories and had started solving the world's problems. During the process one of my buddies, a dentist, commented about how most of the world's leaders ought to see a psychiatrist. From there it was but a six-inch putt to begin the put-down game. We had already trashed lawyers and politicians. So it was inevitable that we trashed the psychiatrists who charge a nominal egg (this is how I heard the phrase "an arm and a leg" when I was in grade school).

The biggest complaint was the money psychiatrists charged for just listening to you babble on about your childhood.

I got on my soapbox and said something like this:

Even if by babbling on and on you came to some understanding as to what happened in your childhood that might be responsible for your current self-destructive character traits or feelings, how does that help? Isn't that the same as finding out that you contracted Trench Mouth from a drinking fountain? That information won't help you now. Knowing causation is of no help unless you're already cured and you want to prevent a recurrence.

Treatment, treatment, treatment. This is what somebody who is sick needs, not just talk, talk, talk. Diagnosis is nice. But diagnosis without treatment is useless to the patient no matter how lucrative it may be to the doctor. I have yet to meet a person who has been "cured" by going to a psychiatrist. Oh, I'm sure that there has to be some success stories. It's just that I haven't met any. I don't think psychiatrists are really that interested in helping people change. They're more interested in finding out what makes them tick than in defusing their personal time bomb.

It was then that one of my opponents whose wife I later found out was a psychiatrist really challenged me. "Okay, Mr. Know-it-all," he sneered, "How do you propose that psychiatrists treat a patient?"

For a split second I almost lost my cool. The phrase, "Mr. Know-it-all" and the tone in his voice pissed me off. I felt like saying, "Listen, you son of a bitch, don't use that tone of voice with me unless you want to end up flat on your ass." But then it occurred to me in a flash. His **words** "Mr. Know-it-all" precipitated his sneer. If you don't believe me, just try to address anybody with that term in a respectful tone and demeanor. Anyway, the words, "Mr. Know-it-all," his tone of voice, and the sneer in turn rattled my cage and an attitude immediately followed. If I had used the words that popped into my mind, I'm sure they would have led to a confrontation. Suddenly, everything fell into place.

> The way a person feels helps determine what he says and the way he says it. What a person says and the way he says it helps determine the way he feels. If you can keep your cool, you can control what you say. If you can control what you say, you can keep your cool.

Of course, that isn't in real scholarly language. If I were writing for a scholarly journal I would have to write something like this:

> Emotional states trigger specific and predictable speech patterns (verbal and non-verbal) that are developed over time. These speech patterns in turn trigger the specific emotional or mental states associated with them.

"So what has this got to do with psychiatrists?" he asked.

"Simple. As long as a psychiatrist's patients continue to use the same language that is associated with whatever particular mental or emotional state that bothers them, these patients will continue exhibiting their problems no matter how well they understand the etiology."

Because I chose to use a conciliatory yet authoritative tone of voice that was not condescending, the incident passed. I didn't continue explicating my theory. We got onto more interesting topics, such as "Did you hear the one about the lawyer, the psychiatrist, and the pickpocket?"

Back home I began to put my ideas down on paper. Suddenly, I realized I had been using these concepts when I was working at the Alternative Junior High School. I remembered the posters that my good friend the art teacher at Northwestern made for me to illustrate the following concept:

Language like clothes
should fit the person
and the occasion.

That clothes should fit the person is fairly easy to illustrate. Picture little Danny DeVito wearing a tuxedo tailor-made for Arnold Swartzennegger. Picture Arnold Swartzenegger wearing a wedding veil, a mini-skirt, combat boots, and holding a baby's rattle in one hand and a lollipop in the other.

That language should fit the person is a little more difficult to illustrate. But picture a supreme court justice using baby talk, a four-year-old expounding on the existentialism in the writings of Feodor Dovstoyeski, an Oriental speaking with an Irish brogue, Rush Limbaugh with a Cockney accent, the Queen of England with a Southern drawl, etc.

That clothes should fit the occasion is fairly easy to illustrate. You don't wear a tuxedo to work on a car. You don't wear dirty grimy overalls to a formal dinner. Basketball players don't wear football uniforms—although maybe they should wear helmets with face masks. There is no one type of dress that fits all occasions. Even blue jeans and tennis shoes can be unacceptable attire.

That language should fit the occasion is a little more difficult to illustrate. But picture a U.S. Marine drill sergeant saying to his troops, "Would you gentlemen kindly stand stiffly erect keeping your feet together and your hands at your side and maintain silence while I am addressing you." Or picture a lawyer using baby talk to a judge, "Oh, your precious little honor, you're so cute. I'm sure you understand why I must make an objection to what the learned counsel just said."

In my first rough draft of this autobiography, I stated rather emphatically that there is no word that in and of itself is objectionable.

In the margin one of my proof readers wrote, "What about the word n----r?"

My answer to that is simple. If you happen to be what today's political correctness calls an African-American, it can be used in a wide variety of instances. For example, I believe that *Nigger* is a highly appropriate word when used by Dick Gregory as the title to his autobiography. In his foreword written to his mother he tells her not to get upset when she hears that word because "...they're just advertising my book." Of course, when a member of any other ethnic group uses that word, it is considered highly inappropriate.

Part of my concept is that words can trigger specific and predictable speech patterns. These speech patterns in turn trigger specific emotional states and behaviors associated with them. Just how accurate this is was illustrated by my daughter's reaction to this sentence from the rough draft of my inservice book, *Get out of my face! Get offa my case!..*

> ### Warning #1
> For reasons you will understand later on, I refuse to use politically correct phrases. If you are a "femi-nazi" ...

She didn't even finish the sentence which read:

> ...you probably will not like my using just *he, his,* and *him*.

She screamed at me, "Dad! You can't use that word! It's obscene!"

I tried to calm her down but by telling her she was proving my point, her fury increased. Even though my wife and I had traveled all the way from Michigan to visit her in California, she threatened to throw me out of her house!

It took her a while to get over her fit of pique and to finish reading the warning which ended with:

If you could be labeled a c---- j-----, c-----, ch---, d---, f---, g---, h----, k---, l----, m---, p----, n-----,

r-----, sp---, w------, w--, yankee or damnyankee, you probably are experiencing right now an emotional reaction to these labels. And if you're a member of one or more of at least a thousand other groups I didn't name but who have labels just as nasty, you still might be reacting negatively to these words. If so, then I should be able to rest my case—but I won't.

It should be self-evident to you that the reasons why you believe that we should attempt to purge sexist or racist language from our everyday speech are the same reasons why we should:

- first identify

- and then modify those words and phrases that create problems for ourselves, the individuals we deal with, and those around us and around them.

The following are eight basic types of speech patterns:

		Negative (Trouble-Making)	Positive (Trouble-Avoiding)
1.	Attention Grabbers	Hey,	Excuse me,
2.	Address	Man,	Mr. McCabe,
3.	Demand vs Request	Take off your *&#!+* hat	If you don't mind, would please remove your hat so I can see.
4.	Emphatics	*&#!+*	_____
5.	Negators	Yeah, but... Like hell, bull shit, No way,	I agree with just about every thing you said except...

6. Defense-Attack	You never...	I don't recall
	Why do you always...?	I wish you ... wouldn't...
	When are you going to stop ...	It bothers me when you start...
	You make me	I find it hard to...
7. Accusatory epithets	Liar!	That's not the way I recall it
	Bitch,	Honey, ...
8. Value Judgments	That's stupid	That's one of the more...

When I give inservices and workshops on this concept, I have the participants fill in the blanks. For example, the phrase, 'You never..." could be filled in with:

> told me that.
> said that I had to...
> take me anywhere.
> buy me anything.
> let me finish what I'm saying.

We also brainstorm and list other phrases that can have blanks to be filled in such as: You're always...(picking on me, late, getting in trouble...)

What becomes clear to my workshop participants is that when a person chooses to use a negative pattern it does four things:

1. It establishes a negative reaction mode in the person speaking.
2. It triggers a negative reaction mode in the person spoken to.
3. It creates specific types of negative self-images and negative self-fulfilling prophecies.
4. It functions as psychic antibodies that kill off invading ideas that teachers, therapists, or counselors may try to use to bring about positive change.

An example that I used in discussing these ideas with Doris Suciu, a leading advocate for helping battered women, was that I really doubt that a man has ever struck his wife without first using that magic word, "Bitch!" Whatever it was that caused his anger in the first place triggers the word "Bitch!" By saying the word "Bitch!" this in turn increases the flow of anger and releases him from normal psychic responsibility. A man doesn't say, "Darling, Honey, or Sweetheart," and then haul off and slug his wife. However, in our society, there's an unspoken code that allows men (and women) to strike out at bitches, bastards, and rectal orifices.

Doris gave me a few other names men use before hitting their wife, none of which I would include in this book.

But there is a brighter side to the picture. If a person's negative speech patterns are identified, with a conscious effort on the person's part and by specifically chosen people surrounding him/her the patterns can either be:

(1) modified,

(2) reduced,

(3) or eliminated by substituting appropriate positive habitual speech patterns which will allow traditional therapeutic measures to work.

For example, if a person has been constantly using the word **never** as the second word in a sentence and he is sensitized to this word, he may consciously start to change what once were automatic patterns that cause confrontations to ones that are more conciliatory. Examples of the negative never sentences are:

1.   You never said that.
2.   You never told me to do that.
3.   I never saw that word before in my life.
4.   I never heard that word before.

Sentences 1 and 2 immediately put the person saying it in a position where he must defend himself from the person he is attacking as a

"LIAR" and who is sure to retaliate at least verbally with something like "Are you calling me a liar?"

Sentences 3 and 4 give the person saying it a clear cut rationalization for not learning that word. How important could it be to learn a specific word if in all a person's previous years of life it hasn't been encountered? The person it is said to intuitively understands that logic but generally doesn't know how to handle it.

Notice that if a substitute phrase such as "I don't recall" is followed by "hearing you say that" or "you telling me to do that," or "seeing that word" or "hearing that word," it cannot truly be disputed. And it doesn't challenge the person who hears it.

As long as the major ways young Americans learn language patterns are from what they hear in the street and on television, we probably shall remain the most violent nation in the world. I believe we should teach those language patterns (including body language patterns) in our schools that tend to help people get along with each other without constantly having confrontations.

Part III, Chapter 22

The Frustrations of trying to find an organization willing to accept a multi-million dollar bequest

YOU WOULD THINK IT would be easy to find a non-profit 501(C)3 organization willing to accept a multi-million dollar bequest. But it isn't, if you happen to be a dyslexic by the name of Don McCabe and you want to ensure that your discoveries about the treatment of dyslexia aren't lost. And one thing for sure that McCabe knows about Murphy's law, is that Murphy is an optimist.

I started the search back in 1989 as the result of convincing the board of directors of the AVKO Foundation that we really should go out of existence in 1999. We started in 1974 and after 25 years if we haven't achieved our simple goals, we don't deserve to stay anyway. And what were our goals? Simple.

1. To determine what it is about the English language that causes so many problems for so many students trying to learn to read and spell it. Our finding: There are not just two types of words, those with regular phonic patterns and those that are irregular. Rather, there are five basic types of spelling. See *English Spelling: The "Simple," the "Fancy," the "Insane," the "Tricky," and the "Scrunched up."* And this is what is so confusing to so many people learning to read English.

2. To determine if all the elements necessary to achieve mastery of reading and spelling English are taught. Our findings: A resounding NO!

3. If there are elements necessary to achieve mastery of reading and spelling English that are not being taught, is it because they can't be taught or because the educational establishment doesn't know that they need to be taught. Our findings: The educational establishment doesn't know (or want to know) that these elements must be taught. The current fad in educational philosophy is that it is best for all students to learn what needs to be learned naturally on their own through the process of whole language instruction.

4. To determine whether or not those who haven't learned (because they haven't been taught) can learn *if* taught properly. Our findings: YES, YES, YES. We have yet to meet a dyslexic that can't be taught to read and spell competently! Yes, we know that somewhere there has to be someone who can't be taught, but McCabe and AVKO just hasn't encountered that someone yet. And we have only encountered a relatively small number of those who just *won't* be taught.

Maybe it's because I'm a dyslexic and have to have things neatly organized that I decided it would take five years to identify the right non-profit to which to give our assets. I also figured that it would take about another five years to make a smooth transition. So we announced our decision to begin the search in our newsletter which was widely disseminated. Shortly thereafter we were contacted by Ohio State University. A group of five instructors flew up from Columbus to Flint in the university's airplane. They took a tour of the foundation and had dinner with some members of the AVKO board at the Frankenmuth Bavarian Inn. They seemed to be impressed. One of the professors seemed to enjoy using the phrase that beautiful gestalt to the materials. He used it over and over. And it's true that there is an underlying unity to the AVKO materials (or gestalt) as the professor put it. They left with smiles on their faces. In about a week I received a letter saying that Ohio State University would be willing to take everything AVKO has right then, lock, stock, and bank accounts. But we had only thirty days in which to do it!

We couldn't believe it. They were giving *us* a deadline!? Obviously we weren't in that much of a rush to deed everything over to Ohio State University with no commitments on their part.

At the next board meeting we had in attendance the treasurer of the Orton Dyslexia Society, the president of Michigan Literacy, Inc., and the president of the Reading Reform Foundation. Again we explained to them our position. We want to go out of existence and leave our assets to an organization that would continue our work and not let it disappear. They nodded their heads. They even posed for a picture. But nothing came of it. We received a letter from the Orton Society respectfully declining to even consider the offer. A month or so later the president of the Learning Disabilities Association of America and the president of the Michigan Learning Disabilities Association visited the foundation as our guests and received the same basic show-and-tell.

They were polite and even affable. But it was thanks but no thanks. Like the others, they didn't want to become involved. If everything we had could be quickly converted to cash they might be interested in it. If it meant helping AVKO get more exposure so that a large publisher would buy the copyrights and pay AVKO (AND ITS HEIRS!) royalties, they didn't want any part of it.

The International Reading Association didn't even bother to answer any of our letters. But then again, they are so large and so well heeled, a few extra millions wouldn't be worth any real effort on their part to try to get.

Part IV – Suggestions to public or private school systems (or home-schoolers) interested in providing the best possible instruction in the basics of reading and writing to all their students.

Part I dealt with my education from birth through college.

Part II covers the period in which my real education began. It will also explain why the materials and techniques I developed to teach dyslexics could not possibly be developed in a traditional academic method.

Part III covers the techniques and materials that I developed because of my own dyslexic symptoms and outlook, techniques and materials that work.

Part IV covers my objections to current reading "theory" and methods of developing reading and spelling programs that will work.

Part IV, Chapter 23

Start your own bandwagon.
Don't just jump on the popular one, especially when they don't know where they're going. Organize your own reading/writing curriculum using measurable minimum standards of achievment.

THERE ARE SEVERAL POPULAR bandwagons available for school systems to jump onto. And many have. One of the more popular is whole language. If you have ever heard one of its major advocates speak, you know it sounds like the answer to every educator's dream. If I don't repeat to you all the theory, it's because I don't want to convince you that this is the bandwagon to jump on. The arguments for using whole language are compelling. But... Always that *but*. Whole language is not working. But that does not stop the theorists from promoting it. That whole language isn't working, isn't the fault of the theory, you see. It's the fault of the teachers who haven't been properly inserviced or if they have been properly inserviced, just don't follow the teachings properly.

Invented spelling is often a component of the whole language approach. That's where students are encouraged to write before they know how to spell, so this way they can invent their own spellings. The teachers don't correct their students' invented spellings because it might hurt their self-esteem. Am I ever glad they didn't encourage invented spelling when I was in school. I can just see a paper written by me describing what I got for Christmas posted on the bulletin board. Sanna brot me a noo (*shirt* spelled without the letter *r*) fir kissmuss.

But before you decide one way or another about invented spelling, let's see what the experts[1] on both sides say:

For	Against
●. Helps bridge the gap between oral and written language for children in early grades.	● Is another example of the "dumbing down" of education.
●. Encourages early, creative writing because children don't have to worry about correct spelling.	● Develops bad language habits at a formative age that are hard to break.
● De-emphasizes memorizing words in favor of under-standing their meaning.	● Discourages formal vocabulary lists and regular spelling tests that make children accountable.
● Builds self-confidence and passion for writing while working up to correct spelling	● Sends children a message that they're never wrong under the guise of making them feel good about their creativity.

Who's right? Would you believe that both sides are right? Ask either side, and they'll tell you. They're right. And I agree. Well, not 100%, and certainly not 110%. What is really wrong, is that neither side can understand the other's point of view.

For a moment let's analyze both sides in reference to establishing some criteria upon which to base our decisions as to what should be in our reading/writing curriculum.

● *Invented spelling helps bridge the gap between oral and written language for children in early grades.*

Question: Is "invented"spelling the *only* way to bridge the gap? Or is it possible that a centuries old technique of dictation used by the French to teach French and by the Russians to teach Russian[2] might

---

[1]Ron Russell, *The Detroit News*, Sunday, March 5, 1995, p. 8A.

[2]This method I mentioned earlier was for me, a dyslexic, the most helpful of all the techniques used at the Army Language School to teach me the Russian language in six months.

accomplish the same thing. And suppose we add the element of immediate student self-correction to dictation, wouldn't that help bridge the gap between oral and written language? And if the dictation were to consist of normal sloppy speech patterns such as, "eye kant bee leave ewe red awl doze store E's" but having the children correctly spell, "I can't believe you read all those stories."

If we taught spelling through dictation as a bridge from oral speech to written, it would definitely not be another example of the "dumbing down" of education.

● *Invented spelling encourages early, creative writing because children don't have to worry about correct spelling.*

I just wonder how many Ernest Hemingways and Dorothy Parkers our country needs. I have nothing against creative writing. At the same time I don't believe that our goal in education should be to encourage creative writing before a child has sufficient knowledge of the world around him and sufficient knowledge of his language to creatively express himself. I do agree that children shouldn't have to **worry** about making mistakes. For years, I have contended that mistakes are opportunities to learn. I have preached that spelling is best taught with a system in which each student gets to *immediately* correct his/her own mistakes. Another benefit of students correcting their mistakes is that in order to correct the mistakes using the dictation method, the student gets practice reading speech patterns converted by the teacher to writing patterns on the chalkboard and on their own paper. All modalities of learning are involved in this method: **A**udio—The student hears the language and hears the spelling of the words—**V**isual. The student sees the correct spelling of the words he has heard the teacher say and sees his own spelling and compares. **K**inesthetic—The student writes the proper letters in the proper sequences. **O**ral—The student says the words and the letters that make up the words.

If that is done, good language habits (not bad) are made at a formative age which helps them achieve the automaticity in spelling necessary for composition in later years.

● *Invented Spelling de-emphasizes memorizing words in favor of understanding their meaning.*

If by de-emphasizing memorizing words we mean de-emphasizing the rote memorization of the spellings, I can't agree more with the intention. To memorize the spellings of words the same way we might memorize telephone numbers is really an irrational approach. But is invented spelling the only way to de-emphasize rote memorization? I think not.

The sequential spelling technique is one that virtually eliminates memorizing. It even eliminates studying! And it works. I cannot, however, agree that invented spelling favors understanding the meanings of the words. It merely allows children to use words whose meanings they *already* know but whose spellings they don't.

As I was writing this section, one of my proofreaders (a dyslexic, himself) reminded me that I used the invented spelling technique with him. Well, yes and no. When I had him write, and remember he was sixteen not six at the time, I encouraged him to use the words he wanted to use not just the words he can spell, because that was another way for me to find words he needed to know how to spell. But I really wasn't using the invented spelling technique. I asked him to just rapidly put down the first few letters that he thought were in the word and then squiggle the rest of the word so it would be about as long as he envisioned it to be. I didn't want him to fixate on the spelling of any one word. However, as soon as he had finished his composition, we corrected it. His misspellings were not left standing. His misspellings, cute as some of them may have been, were not exhibited for others to see and enjoy at his expense.

Another bandwagon is the *"Hooked on Phonics."* I generally do not like to just out and out trash a commercial product. So, I won't. I'll only say that I was immediately dubious about its claims, but unlike most reading experts, I wouldn't say anything about it until I had purchased a set for the AVKO Educational Research Foundation, examined it, and had some students use it. We have *Hooked on Phonics*. We will lend it out to anyone. So far no one we have lent it to has finished it. But I am sure that somewhere someone has had success with it.

Am I in favor of teaching phonics? If by that you mean am I in favor of having students sit by themselves at their desk and work on dittoed sheets in which they circle short vowels and draw lines over long vowels and cross out silent vowels, then the answer is no. Again, there may be some phonic worksheets that have helped certain students learn specific skills that helped them become good readers. In my personal experience, phonic worksheets are simply tools used by teachers to keep their students busy while they take care of their routine busy work.

Am I in favor of students *learning* phonics? Well, I have yet to meet a good reader who didn't know his phonics. By this I mean, a good reader can automatically read non-words such as incordation, cligging, cleacher, and supercandidnaciously as well as "Mistuh Kint Clah'k be a fixin' to ax you sumthin 'bout yor innerestin' life stowry." That same reader might not be able to recite the rules about open and closed vowels and when you double a consonant and when you don't. But so what? If a reader responds to the conventions of spelling so that he hears what the writer intends, then, from a practical standpoint, he knows his phonics.

And this is just one of the many things that we as educators should strive to do. That is, we should strive to make sure all our students can pronounce almost any real word or nonsense word by the time they finish the eighth grade.

Before we can achieve this goal, we must:

1. know exactly what are all our spelling conventions,

2. make sure that the curriculum specifically teaches all the conventions, not just the most frequently used words.

At the time I am writing this sentence, March 14, 1995, I do not believe that there is a single curriculum coordinator in any school system in the United States who can list or find a list of our spelling conventions. I also believe that there is not a single person in any of the state or federal departments of education who can locate such a list.

Is there such a list? Would I ask that question if I didn't know the answer? Of course, there is a list. It the list of patterns that I used to make sure that my Sequential Spelling Series covered every single pattern. It is the list of patterns that helped me put together the nearly 1,000 pages of the *Patterns of English Spelling.* I have it, and I want to share it. Perhaps by the year 2,000 there may be some educational leaders who not only know of its existence but are using it to ensure that all students have the opportunity of having these patterns presented to them so that they can learn them. Less than 1/3 of all the spelling patterns are taught in our schools. Less than 5% of all the words we use in daily life are taught in schools. Is it any wonder we are experiencing such wide spread illiteracy?

Yet I have faith that teachers can teach all their students who want to learn how to read and how to spell. What our teachers need the most is to be told *what* it is they have to teach and just *what* their students must demonstrate that they have learned.

What I propose is that public or private school systems (or home-schoolers) interested in providing the best possible instruction in the basics of reading and writing to all their students first evaluate their present spelling program. This is a relatively simple thing to do. But not so simple that I will take time out here to explain it. Yet, not so complex that I will leave it out. You can find the method in the appendix under the title: *How to Evaluate Your Present Spelling Program.*

The next step is to have a spelling curriculum committee sit down and hammer out a specific listing of which spelling patterns are to be systematically taught in which grade. Generally speaking, the words containing the simple patterns will be taught in the first three grades. The advanced and the fancy patterns such as "shuss" being spelled -

cious as in suspicious will be taught in the later grades. Perhaps the most difficulty will be encountered with the teaching of homophones and homographs, the tricky words such as *read/reed/red/read.* There are perhaps fifty times as many in our language as are really taught. Most of the elementary teachers won't want to teach insane words such as *rendezvous, résumé, solder, colonel,* and *lingerie.* Yet they need to be taught. And the scrunched up words? We really "hafta" teach these and the best way is through sentence dictation in which the students minds are temporarily focusing on spelling one or two specific words in the sentence and not the "have to" as in the sentence: *You have to expect an exception or two once in a while.* All the time your target for mastery is *"hafta"* correctly spelled as *have to.* Using daily dictation sentences (and that could be in almost every class where pencils and paper are used) all varieties of spelling patterns, including the insane, will normally be covered.

But for this to happen, it will take some doing to get the schools to change. Why? Well, when it comes to change, it seems that school systems are damned if they do and damned if they don't. Perhaps, rightfully so. It seems that when it comes to buying up-to-date textbooks in history and science, many school systems just can't find enough money in the budget. But when it comes to subjects in which there is little or no change, they find the money to buy books on "new" math where concepts are more important than right answers and kids can use calculators without learning their multiplication tables. We can find English transformational grammar books with "trees of derivation" and "proof" that English has only two tenses, past and present. No future tense in English. What will our university professors think of next?

And when it comes to buildings and classrooms, we keep designing new and better monstrosities. Schools with gymnasiums in the center built on swamp land so that the walls crack as the building settles in the first year. Remember, I taught in one of those. I also taught in one that had air-conditioning that worked only when all the classroom doors were closed. The engineers, architects, and administrators who approved the design had forgotten that every hour for five minutes every single classroom door opens for class change. I have even tried to teach in a school that had no walls separating classrooms. Open classrooms! Somehow that was supposed to be the answer. It isn't.

Then we come to curriculum changes. We threw out phonics over sixty years ago along with diagramming and parsing and went to sight methods of teaching reading. Dick and Jane and controlled vocabulary within basal readers were going to lead us to the promised land of 100% literacy. Lately, the gurus in the universities began looking for something new to use. They had been defending their sight methods of teaching by attacking phonics for so long, that any return to any form of phonics was out of the question. They found what they wanted in New Zealand of all places. Whole language! Invented spelling! What's next in the step backwards towards total illiteracy? Invented letters? Was Dr. Seuss ahead of his time with his *On Beyond Zebra*?

But don't think I'm criticizing Dr. Seuss. By no means. His books *should* be taught in schools. In fact, I have used his book *The Sneetches* to teach the concepts of allegory symbolism, and satire to college students! His books are fun to read. His books have moral tales just like Aesop's fables. They have rhyme. They have rhythm. But according to the college professor who at least considers herself the eminent authority in kiddy lit, Seuss's books are just too much fun for kids to read in class. If the kids want them, let them buy them or go to the library and check them out. Just don't teach them. The same went for Jan and Stan Berenstain's Bear books. They're fun. They're great for beginning readers. But for some reason, most of the books that are fun books just don't fit into the whole language approach. The whole language approach is supposed to make students appreciate *literature*. So they have the little kids analyze the stories, draw webs, make plot lines, do character analysis. Ugh. It's no wonder most students don't read novels for fun.

Now, as I have said before, there are elements of the whole language approach that are sound. Good teachers have used those principles for years. But the whole language band wagon has not worked and will not work. And how about the return to basics band wagon? Well, if I had to choose between the two, I suppose I would take the back to basics—but reluctantly. Why? Because the leaders of this movement don't understand the basics themselves, at least in regards to the spelling patterns of our language. They don't understand the phonics of our language, although they think they do.

The phonics taught even by the best approaches which use multi-sensory techniques still miss the mark. What they teach enables students to spell fisherman as *fishermun* or *fishurmun* and *precious* as *preshus*. They teach single letter sound correspondences going from left to right. Does that work?

Well, pronounce each of the following words and note where the changes occur:

ma   mag   magi   magic   magician

Al   ale   (t)alk   all   allow   alm

Ma	Letter a is pronounced "AH"
mag	Letter a is short as in apple. Letter g is hard.
Magi	Letter a is short as in apple. Letter g is soft ("J"). The letter i is long.
magic	Letter a is short. Letter g is soft ("J"). The letter i is short. The letter c is pronounced /k/.

magician	Letter a is now "uh." The letters ici are pronounced "ish." The letters -an are pronounced "un" —not "AN" as in man, tan, and pan.
Al	a=short a as in pal, Hal, Sal, gal
ale	a="AY" as in pale, hale, male, female
alk	al="AW" as in talk, walk, chalk, stalk
all	al="AW" as in fall, ball, wall, tall
allow	a="uh" as in allowance, allowed
alm	al="AH" as in palm, calm, psalm, qualms

Does this mean our language isn't phonic? Not at all. It is about 99% perfectly phonic if you consider the patterns that letters make, not individual letters themselves. For example: Let's work backward from the word *magician*. The -an ending is always pronounced "un" and it nearly always carries the meaning of a hum*an* whether an American, Canadian, Mexican, Russian, or fireman. When the *-an* is preceded by the letters *ci* the *cian* is always pronounced "shun" and again carries the meaning of a human that makes whatever the -ic word was, as in a *musician* makes *music*, a *magician* makes *magic*, and a *physician* can give you a *physic* (Trust me, you really don't want one) or a *physical* and, of course, an *electrician* makes anything *electrical* such as an *electric* motor correctly use *electricity*.

Back to ma, mag, magi, magic and magician. When the letter i comes after the letter g , the letter usually makes the letter g sound as a /j/. When a word ends with the letter i it usually is either a long i or a long ee as in magi or macaroni.

Although the sound of the letter a changes in the -al+ words, the sounds of any total pattern is consistent. For example, all the -alk words rhyme with hawk. All the -all words rhyme with crawl.

Some more consistencies are: When a short one syllable word ends in g preceded by any vowel, the g is hard as in bag, beg, big, bog, and bug. When a one syllable word ends with the letter a, the a never is short. For example, da, fa, ha, la, ma, and pa. If you add the letter t to any of those words, notice that they will all rhyme with bat and cat and rat. What is consistent in our language are the patterns within words—not the individual letter-sound correspondences. These consistencies can be taught. They shouldn't be left for the students to learn by themselves. Which, by the way, all good readers have done. They have learned them. They weren't taught these patterns. But nevertheless they learned them, despite the methods of reading instruction that they received.

The band wagon I would want you to create is a simple enough one.

> Let's teach the spelling patterns
> that are used to make the words
> we use for reading and writing.

But what about the dialects of English? Over and over I have heard the opponents of any phonics approach scream that question. And never listen to the answer. They think that by asking the question, they have totally destroyed any argument for teaching the sounds of our language. Wrong!

What American schools need to do is to teach a wider variety of American (and British) English languages so that all Americans can communicate with each other in at least the standard TV and radio dialect as well as their own and perhaps one or two more.

It doesn't really matter what particular non-TV or radio dialect one has. The further away from that TV dialect that one speaks, the less likely the person is to achieve what is usually perceived to be a successful position in our business world, Ross Perot being the exception to prove the rule.

So what I propose is to have a band wagon to teach our TV-Radio dialect as a second language to all students as well as teaching others to understand enough other dialects so that they know that the sound of "SIT da-oun ratcheer" is merely "Sit down right here" and that "Rock eel" is not a fish but rather a city in NAWTH Carolina spelled Rock Hill.

We don't have to label any non-standard dialect as anything except non-standard. If a student wants to say he has been "a fixin' to ax me tuh do sumpthin," that's perfectly all right as long as the situation doesn't call for standard TV-Radio dialect. In which case, the student should be able to speak correctly and tell me he "has been planning to ask me something." Generally speaking, most conversations in schools should be conducted in standard TV-Radio dialect. Most students get sufficient practice in their local dialect at home and in the streets.

So, you might say the band wagon I would want you to create is the give every child the bi-lingual phonic patterns approach to English reading and spelling. The ability to speak and write standard American TV-Radio dialect should be a pre-requisite for nearly every teacher. More important than the band wagon itself, is the direction it should be going in. Unless we know where we want to go and what is necessary to get there, a band wagon is not enough. A good map is a help. Knowledge of the roads, their conditions, the rivers and bridges or fords come in handy. And so is a compass.

How do we determine where we want to go? Well, first we might ask for input from members of our community as to what they believe every high school student should be able to do. See the sample Survey Form on the next page.

		Sample Survey Form
Yes	No	
___	___	Should every high school graduate be able to read and spell every word in this short survey form? If no, which words would you allow a student to miss reading? Which words would you allow a graduating high school senior to misspell, and how badly?
___	___	Should every student be able to both print and write legibly?
___	___	Should every student be able to speak in standard American TV-Radio dialect so that his/her particular dialect does not pose an obstacle to achieving success.
___	___	Should every student know how to behave in social situations that demand specific behaviors. For example, should they exhibit knowledge of what type of body language, dress code, and dialect would be appropriate in a court appearance, for a job interview, at a family reunion, or in a neighborhood hangout?

Naturally I would prefer you to make your own lists of questions. But if you decide to use my sample survey form, it means that you should test at least a sizable sampling of your school system's population to determine if most of them can read it. And spell it from dictation.

I doubt very much that many high school principals or school superintendents would want this survey form dictated to their students. Why? Because they wouldn't want the taxpayers who are supporting their school to see just how badly their students spell. The chances are that less than 5% would be able to correctly spell all the words in that very simple survey. Chances are that over half would misspell at least ten words! After writing this, I gave this test to the first high school students I met. One was an "honor roll" student. The following are just some of their misspellings:

Student A	Student B	Student C
graduet	grajuit	graduat
serway	sirway	
seaner		senor
legably	legiblely	ligebly
standerd		
obstical	obsatcle	abstocle
	acheiveing	acheiving
susces		sussess
poppyulayshun	popolation	
prinsipals	principles	prinsiples
duturmin		deturmin
	soshal	sociel
sitchuations	situtations	
spasific		spesifick

behavors	*behaveurs*	*behaviers*
	exibit	
	knowlege	*nolej*
apropreit	*aporperiat*	*aporpiet*
	apearence	*appearance*
intervue		
	reunoin	
naberhood		*nieghborhood*

Organizing your own reading/writing curriculum using measurable minimum standards of achievement.

It's not enough to have a long list of nice sounding generalities such as 75% of the student body will be reading within one grade level of the grade they are in as measured by Brand X Reading Comprehension Test. How can you ensure it? Besides, you could have 25% of your student body be totally illiterate and still achieve your goal. Or what's even worse, is for a school to set a ridiculously low target goal such as 26% of the student body reaching minimum goals. This the Detroit Public Schools did in 1994. True, it was an increase of 2% over the previous year.[1] Yet, to congratulate yourself, as the Detroit Public Schools did, in their annual report for having achieved their previous goal (24% of their students reading adequately) is a shameful and deceitful practice. The goal that they had reached with the 24% was an increase over the previous 21%.

Perhaps the most difficult of all pitfalls to avoid in setting goals and assessing students, is the reading comprehension trap. No, I'm not against reading comprehension. And I'm not against God, our country, our flag, and motherhood. But I am dead set against using

---

[1]Detroit Public Schools 1993-1994 Annual Report, p. 21.

tests that assume something to be true which isn't. Would anyone dare to publish audio tapes that purported to test listening comprehension if the tapes had obvious distortions in sound, breaks in sound, and bits of static all through it? Of course not. But that is exactly what a reading comprehension test is to a student who cannot decode (pronounce correctly) all the words.

Reading comprehension tests *assume* 100% correct decoding by those taking the test.

Less than 100% correct decoding means that incorrect answers are caused, not by the lack of the ability to comprehend, but by the lack of the ability to correctly "hear" because of the "static."

First things first. Before reading comprehension tests are given and scored, students should be able to read all the words. Then, all the words used should be within their vocabulary—if we are truly testing *comprehension*. Would you like to stake your reputation of understanding what you read on this "simple" little reading comprehension test?

Oswald made both hands. First he squeezed me. Then he squeezed my partner. On the next board, he stripped the hand. Then he made a simple end play.

1. Oswald is most likely a member of:
A—ACLU; B—NAACP; C—ACBL; D—UAW

2. Oswald in the story is my:
A—friend; B—father; C—opponent; D— partner

3. Oswald's last name is most likely:
A—Smith; B—Owens; C—Jacoby; D—Churchill

Chances are that you could get the first two questions right using the process of elimination. You may not know what the paragraph is about, but you know it doesn't have anything to do with civil liberties, so you can eliminate the ACLU (American Civil Liberties Union). As race doesn't seem to play any part, you can eliminate the National Association for the Advancement of Colored People (NAACP). Labor doesn't seem to play a part so you can eliminate the United Auto Workers (UAW). That leaves just the ACBL. The second question is easy enough to infer that if Oswald wasn't my partner, he was most likely my opponent. But even if you scored 67% correct, do you really have any comprehension?

As I am writing this, I realized that had I had given this test last night to the 28 people I was with, they would have all scored 100% correct. Why? Not because the readability is below the third grade level, but because they were all members of the American Contract Bridge League (ACBL). They all use the terms "hand" to describe the 13 cards they are dealt, "board" for the metal holder the "hands" are put into after being dealt. They all would immediately recognize the duplicate bridge situation and know that Oswald would be my opponent. And because the name of Oswald Jacoby is as famous in the bridge world as Michael Jordan is in the basketball world, they would automatically get all the answers right.

In order to be sure that you answer a reading comprehension question correctly, you must:

1. be able to read all the words,
2. know what the words mean,
3. know the meaning within the context of the selection.
4. apply related knowledge.

So first things first. Schools should insist that students be able to correctly decode 99.5% of all words they encounter. Good readers correctly decode at least 99.9% of the words they encounter. Surely, in this book which has approximately 350 words per page, there shouldn't be more than 1.75 words per page that a good reader cannot read. 99.5% efficiency in reading text is not unreasonable.

Vocabulary is next in importance. And vocabulary is rarely systematically taught even though the leaders in the field of education have known for years that the best single predictor of success in college is a simple 25 word vocabulary test.

So? If a school system wants literate graduates, the first thing they must do is to ensure that their students learn to decode words automatically. If they want to very scientifically make their own decoding *tests*, they can have their computer whizzes set up a program that lists all the onsets and rimes. It can randomly produce non-words such as clig, cligging, cliggle, clickle, climple, clestionable, clision, clission, unclissionably, and preclique. This way, if a student can correctly read *clision* to rhyme with *vision*, you can be reasonably sure that he responds automatically to the -ision rime. But if the student reads *preclique* as "preck luh cue" rather than rhyming it with *pree cleek* you can be reasonably sure that he wouldn't be able to read Angelique has a unique boutique in Mozambique.

At the moment there is no listing of all the "rimes" in any of the reference tools used by the major publishers. Why? Well, I guess I have to take the blame for that. I haven't taken the time to pound on their doors and scream in their ears that I have such a tool, that they need such a tool, that they should buy that tool, and that they should allow me to teach them how to use that tool. *Mea culpa, mea culpa, mea maxima culpa.*

If a school system wants to really set its literacy goals by using criteria that can be measured, the AVKO Educational Research Foundation, is willing to help them do it. We can tell you exactly what has to be learned. The school system can determine when each component is to be taught, how it is to be taught, and if it's being learned.

Part III, Chapter 24

What is dyslexia? Official definitions defined.

If it looks like a duck, walks like a duck,
it's probably a duck.
The wrong road that the most current and expensive research on
dyslexia is headed.

A Few Definitions of Dyslexia:

- DYSLEXIA IS: "a disorder manifested by difficulty in learning to read despite conventional instruction, adequate intelligence and sociocultural opportunity."

  —World Federation of Neurology

  > Translation: *If a student isn't dumb and he isn't surrounded by people who hate schools and he goes to school and gets the "conventional instruction" (Look-see or whole language or even phonics), and he has problems reading, it must be that he is dyslexic.*

- Developmental dyslexia is a specific learning disability characterized by difficulty in learning to read. Some dyslexics also may have difficulty learning to write, to spell, and, sometimes, to speak or to work with numbers. We do not know for sure what causes dyslexia, but we do know that it affects children who are physically and emotionally healthy, academically capable, and who come from good home environments. In fact, many dyslexics have the advantages of excellent schools, high mental ability, and parents who are well-educated and value learning.

  —U.S. Department of Health and Human Services

Translation: *We don't know for sure what causes dyslexia, but the difficulty in learning to read, spell, speak, or do math (dyslexia) can affect healthy, intelligent people who attend excellent schools (nice buildings, well paid teachers, and look-see or whole language curriculum) and have a good family environment.*

- Dyslexia is a neurologically-based, often familial, disorder which interferes with the acquisition and processing of language. Varying in degrees of severity, it is manifested by difficulties in receptive and expressive language, including phonological processing, in reading, writing, spelling, handwriting, and sometimes in arithmetic. Dyslexia is not a result of lack of motivation, sensory impairment, inadequate instructional or environmental opportunities, or other limiting conditions, but may occur together with these conditions. Although dyslexia is life-long, individuals with dyslexia frequently respond successfully to timely and appropriate intervention.

—Definition proposed by
Committee of Members
Orton Dyslexia Society , Nov., 1994.

Translation: *This means dyslexia is related to the structure of the brain itself that may either be inherited or caused by brain damage.[1] The bell curve applies to dyslexics as well as all other segments of society in regards to the individual difficulties in understanding language (written, oral, and body) and in using language in speaking or writing. Dyslexia is*

---

[1] My dyslexia could be the result of brain damage. I suffered birth trauma, but since my son and one of my grandsons is dyslexic, it could also be genetic, or perhaps even both.

not the result of a child not trying or not having sufficient motivation. Dyslexia is not the result of something wrong with the eyes or the ears. Dyslexia is not the result of poor teaching or poor environments. Dyslexia cannot be cured. But some dyslexics can be taught to read and write if they receive "proper" teaching early enough.

- Dyslexia is one of several distinct learning disabilities. It is a specific language-based disorder of constitutional origin characterized by difficulties in single word decoding, usually reflecting insufficient phonological processing abilities. These difficulties in single word decoding are often unexpected in relation to age and other cognitive and academic abilities; they are not the result of generalized developmental disability or sensory impairment. Dyslexia is manifested by variable difficulty with different forms of language, often including, in addition to problems reading, a conspicuous problem with acquiring proficiency in writing and spelling.

—Orton Dyslexia Society
Research Committee, Nov. 1994

Translation: Much the same as the other translations.

What is *my* definition of *dyslexia*? I don't bother defining dyslexia. To me, the word *dyslexia* is a word much like the word *love*. We all know what *love* is. But the more we try to define exactly what *love* is and what *love* is not, the more confused we get.

Besides, who cares what the best definition is? All I care about is that everybody should receive proper instruction in reading and writing. As far as I am concerned, *everybody* can be taught to read and write at least as well as they can speak.

But if I am pressed to give a definition of dyslexia, rather than invent one of my own, I think I would choose the one the Orton

Dyslexia Society uses in its brochure *dys✦lex✦ia DEFINING THE PROBLEM*. The following passage is quoted directly from this pamphlet. The only exception is the clearly marked notation concerning my personal traits that are associated with dyslexia.

The word dyslexia is derived from Greek: *dys* (poor or inadequate); and *lexis* (words). The English meaning is poor or inadequate language. Dyslexia is characterized by problems in expressive or receptive, oral or written language. Problems may emerge in reading, spelling, writing, speaking, or listening. Dyslexia is not a disease; it has no cure. Dyslexia describes a different kind of mind—often gifted and productive—that learns differently. Intelligence is not the problem. Dyslexics may have average to superior intelligence. An unexpected gap exists between their learning aptitude and their achievement in school.

The problem is not behavioral. It is not psychological. It is not social. It is not a problem of vision; dyslexics do not "see backward." Dyslexia results from differences in the structure and the function of the brain.

Dyslexics are unique. Each has individual strengths and weaknesses. Many dyslexics are creative and have unusual talent in areas such as art, athletics, architecture, graphics, electronics, mechanics, drama, music, or engineering. Dyslexics often show special talent in areas that require visual, spatial, and motor integration.

Their problems in language processing distinguish them as a group. This means that the dyslexic has problems translating language to thought (as in listening or reading) or in translating thought to language (as in writing or speaking).

—Definition continues on next three pages—

CHARACTERISTICS *that may accompany dyslexia*	*Characteristics* *that I possess*
✓ Lack of awareness of sounds in words—sound order, rhymes, or sequence of syllables.	*When I take tests that use nonsense words run together in normal speech patterns, I fail miserably.*
✓ Difficulty decoding words— single word identification.	*I have no problem. My sister was a good teacher*
✓ Difficulty encoding words —spelling.	*Again, no problem. Same reason*
✓ Poor sequencing of numbers of letters in words, when read or written, e.g.: b-d; p-q, sing-sign; left-felt; soiled-solid; 12-21.	*In tests using nonsense words without normal patterns such as nsoeensn, I do miserably. Transposing numbers has often created problems for me, especially dialing telephone numbers.*
✓ Problems with reading comprehension.	*No real problem. Same reason.*
✓ Difficulty in expressing thoughts orally.	*Yes. I never know when something I know, word or fact or name, suddenly cannot be retrieved. But I have developed many compensating verbal skills.*

CHARACTERISTICS *that may accompany dyslexia*	*Characteristics that I possess*
✓Delayed spoken language.	*I was the slowest in my family to talk. I had speech therapy from 1st Grade through the 4th..*
✓ Imprecise or incomplete interpretation of language that is heard.	*I heard "mustard" for Buster, and "for all intensive purposes" instead of intents and purposes. I find it diffi-cult to hear words when sung or when I can't see the person who is speaking.*
✓Confusion about directions in space or time (right and left, up and down, early and late, yesterday and tomor-row, months and days).	*In buildings or in cities where hallways or streets do not follow nice neat patterns, I'm lost. Without a watch, I have no sense of time.*
✓Confusion about right or left handedness.	*I bat and throw with both hands, and can even write with both hands or play table tennis equally badly with both hands.*
✓Similar problems among relatives.	*My son and grandson exhibit many of the same symptoms.*
✓Difficulty with handwriting	*The only grade below an A that I received in grade school was in handwriting. Although most people*

CHARACTERISTICS *that may accompany dyslexia*	*Characteristics* *that I possess*
	consider my handwriting to be excellent, *I have never achieved what would been* *good enough for my Cook School* *teachers to be worth a grade of B.*
✓Difficulty in mathematics— often related to sequencing of steps or directionality or to the language of mathematics.	*As long as I had good teachers, I* *have had no problem.* *However, learning the symbols and* *formulas in statistics was a* *nightmare for me.*

FEW DYSLEXICS EXHIBIT ALL THE SIGNS OF THE DISORDER. THEIR PROBLEMS IN LANGUAGE PROCESSING DISTINGUISH THEM AS A GROUP.

End of Quotation. *Column* of *italics* is *mine*.

Would I add any characteristics to Orton's list? Yes. Having a logical mind and wanting to know *why* is a characteristic I have found most dyslexics to share. Most dyslexics by the time they reach high school will be able to read and spell *cat, fish, peck,* and *helpful.* Yet a word like *special* is liable to absolutely throw them for a loop. Why? Logic. Major premise. Words with the letter c have either a /k/ sound or a /s/ sound. "Spek•eye•al" is not a word. "Spee•sigh•AL" is not a word. All combinations of sounds and accents lead to nothing. The word *special* can't be sounded out using what I have been **taught**. BEEP BEEP BEEP goes the logical computer. It does not compute. Non-dyslexics generally have no problem learning this word. Logic and rules don't interfere. Someone told them that the letters s-p-e-c-i-a-l spell special. So they learned.

Maybe not the first time, but it didn't take many repetitions for them to learn.

And I do think the problem lies in the underlying, unstated, and definitely not-admitted-to-by-our-educational-leaders assumption that schools need only ensure that students learn the names of the letters of the alphabet, write the letters somewhat legibly, surround the students with words and pretty pictures, and expose them to literature, and they'll learn to read. That this is all that is necessary for some to learn to read is undoubtedly true. And it is some of these "some" who run our schools. Their unspoken logic is: What was enough for them to learn should be good enough for everybody else. WRONG!

What should dyslexia researchers _NOT_ be researching?

1. Who we should blame for dyslexia? Our parents' genes? Our schools? Our language?

2. What should we blame for dyslexia? The brain itself?

The wrong road that the most current and expensive research on dyslexia is headed is just where you might suspect it would be: Number 1 finding the blame. Among the more expensive and stupid research that is being done is being done with cadavers of known dyslexics. Researchers are carefully pickling their brains and slicing them deli-thin and comparing the dyslexic slices with brains from normal cadavers. They hope to demonstrate that there is a difference. I have no doubt they will. Big hairy deal. If the same scientists were to pickle and slice paper thin the leg muscles of paraplegics, and then compare them with paper thin slices of pickled normal human leg muscles, there will be a difference. I wonder why. Might it be that things that are used by the mind or body might differ from those that aren't?

And if after spending millions or billions of dollars, they can determine that the fault is in the brain, so what? How does that knowledge help a single dyslexic? It doesn't.

The same goes for the genetic research that is going on. I listened to the experts put on their dog and pony show at the 94 National Orton Dyslexia Society Conference. They think they have located the genetic marker. Wonderful. After a few more millions spent, they might be able to have a DNA test that could be used to determine if a child is pre-disposed to being dyslexic. Maybe even in the womb! Big deal. Big hairy deal. Just how is that knowledge going to help a single dyslexic? Again, it isn't.

What should dyslexia researchers BE researching?

1. How and when and if we should identify dyslexics?

2. When, how, and with what materials and techniques should we use to teach dyslexics?

Treatment of dyslexia is what is important, not determining who or what is to blame. And identification and labeling of dyslexics? What is important is not stamping a scarlet D for Dumb on a student but rather helping that student. Today, millions are still being spent trying to find ways of early identification. Almost nothing is being spent on finding effective ways of treating kids who can't read and just as importantly, getting these methods and materials into our schools. In fact, the largest and best of all organizations devoted to helping dyslexics, The Orton Dyslexia Society, has as part of its credo—its disclaimer that it will NOT recommend any specific program, school, or materials. Unless Orton and its larger brethren, the International Reading Association, relax their seemingly logical neutral stance of not recommending anything that might work, the giants in the publishing industry have nothing to worry about. They love the status quo. They're making money at it.

But back to identification of dyslexic. Is early identification desirable? Everybody seems to think so. But ask Dr. Eldo Bergman from Houston, Texas just how important it was to identify his son as dyslexic when he was kindergarten. He'll tell you that from the day he knew for sure that his second son was dyslexic, he fought to get the best schooling possible for his son. He did all the right things. He even sent his boy to a private school with class sizes limited to six. He had tutors for his son. And until his son had phonics drilled into him, he was making no gains at all. And even the phonics with the best of Orton Gillingham didn't do the trick.

> ## Early identification of dyslexia is worthless unless effective remediation takes place.

And how much money is being spent on effective remediation? Well, just try to get grant money in this area. It's really impossible. Grants for gimmicks, yes. Grants for studies of existing programs that don't work, yes. Grants for creating new programs, no. Grants for developing materials, no. If you think I'm wrong, please, please prove it to me. Help the AVKO Foundation get some grant money! We're not proud. We'll accept federal, state, local, corporate, or foundation grants. But please don't just say we should have tried harder. If you know how to do it, do it for us. Better yet, do it for a whole nation filled with kids at risk.

One of the things we tried to do many years ago was to get all the major education organizations to jointly apply for funding. As I envisioned it, there would have been two or three competitive research and development programs going on at various major university centers, such as the Center for the Study of Reading at the University of Illinois, the Center for the Study of Teaching at Michigan State University, and the Center for Family Literacy at Indiana University. The major educational publishers would be involved. They would have everything to gain and nothing really to lose by joining in. The government and philanthropic foundations would be footing the bill. The object, of course, would be to find the most efficient and effective ways of ensuring that all students graduate with the ability to read and write—not just the non-dyslexics. Were any organizations interested? Not one answered. Were any of the universities interested? Not one answered. But since the challenge was sent also out to thousands of other educators, I did get some replies. Most of the said about the same thing. "Good luck. You'll need it. But I don't think you can overcome the battles over turf." They were right.

Which comes to the great Catch-22 of reading research. If it is true that "in fact, many dyslexics have the advantages of excellent schools, high mental ability, and parents who are well-educated and value learning" what's the point in trying to develop material for them? They can't learn to read.

Hogwash!

> Dyslexia is as much the result of bad teaching techniques and even worse teaching materials and insane curriculum design as it is the results of various neurological dysfunctions that may be either inherited or results of trauma.

Strong words? Yes. Heresy? Yes. No self-respecting member of the Orton Dyslexia Research Committee would agree to that. But damn it all, it's true. We can pour millions of dollars into building beautiful schools and millions more staffing them with teachers who have Ph.D.'s in Education, and security guards trained in all the martial arts, and we still won't solve the problem.

Do you remember the piece *60 Minutes* did on the Kansas City Schools? Great TV journalism. But saddening. They were spending money on all the wrong things.

Other than Cook School, the best school I ever attended had the least in terms of things physical. Flint Technical had no gym, no library, no auditorium, no cafeteria. Yet it was by far the best high school in the city of Flint as long as it existed. In case you skipped the first part of the book, that story occurs in Chapter 4.

What did Flint Tech have?

● Good teachers,

● a good principal,

● a good curriculum,

● good students and

● good student discipline.

The order is not important. Every element has to be there. Lose one and you might end up losing all the rest.

Part IV, Chapter 25

Common Misconceptions about Dyslexia

Dyslexics see letters backwards. They see b's when they should be seeing d's. Wrong! The image on a dyslexic's retina is the same as that of anybody elses. True, it is upside down. That's normal. Every human is born seeing everything upside down. But it doesn't take long for our computer brains to take its visual sensory input and make it agree with its inner sense of reality by reversing it. You can purchase a special type of goggles that will make you see everything upside down. However, if you wear them long enough, the computer brain once again forces its data into making sense, and even with the reversing vision glasses on, you see rightside up. Of course, the moment you take these glasses off, now you're seeing upside down. But not to worry, the correct vision is fairly quickly restored.

How did this misconception come about? It came about because people working with dyslexics noticed that their students would often read *was* for *saw* and *saw* for *was*. They would write *d*'s for *b*'s and *p*'s for *g*'s or *q*'s. The misconception came about because so many people jumped to the wrong conclusion. The misreading or miswriting came about not because the visual images the dyslexics had in their mind were somehow twisted around, but because of the way the computer brain is pre-programmed to operate.

For example, let's look at four different pictures in which the positioning of the same object makes no difference as to what the object is. But the word being used to illustrate the sound of the letter and the letter itself? Hmmm.

		bird **b**	**b**	**b**
		cup **c**	**c**	**c**
		dish **d**	**d**	**d**
		fish **f**	**f**	**f**

We have a bird, a cup, a dish and a fish. Wonderful. But isn't the next group of pictures, pictures of the same bird, cup, dish, and fish? The idea was to have the person tutoring say to the person learning to read:

This is a bird. Say bird.

This is the letter b inside the bird.

This is the word bird. Say bird.

This is the letter b. Say b.

Although this approach can be demonstrated as an effective tool for most beginning readers, there is a built-in problem. Dyslexics won't remember which way the bird's head is pointing, which way the cup hanging, which side of the plate the spoon is on, or which way the fish is swimming and which way its tail is pointed..

Look at the next group of pictures. Aren't they exactly the same bird, cup, dish, and fish?

d	d	bɹid d		
ɔ	ɔ	qʊɔ ɔ		
b	b	dƨib b		
ɟ	ɟ	dƨiɟ ɟ		

Here we have a bird, a cup, a dish, and a fish. What's next?

If we read left to right, the word bird still starts with a b and ends with a d. But the letter b in the letter column is a d. The p in cup is a q.

But let's look at these letters again another way.

ɟ	ɟ	ɟ **fish**		
p	p	p **dish**		
ɔ	ɔ	ɔ **cup**		
q	q	q **bird**		

Here we have a fish, dish, cup, and bird. But look again.

We have no problem recognizing the objects. But the letters?!

Now the letter in the letter box in front of the bird is a q. The first letter in the word box in front of the dish is a p. Hmm.

So let's look another way.

🐟	🐟	t ɥsıɟ	t	t
🔔	🔔	q qıǝɥ	q	q
🎩	🎩	c cnb	c	c
🐦	🐦	p pɹıq	p	p

By now, it should become quite apparent that the *position* of objects is meaningless to the computer brain. A bird is a bird is a bird no matter what direction its tail or head is pointed. But a **p** or a **d** or a **q** can be associated with a bird's body and tail and consequently interpreted by the dylexic mind as a **b**. Because position is so important for letter recognition and because letter recognition is so important for reading and spelling, initial reading programs that use objects for letter association, can *unintentionally* create *reversal* problems for *dyslexics*.

They need a more kinesthetic approach to letter identification rather than purely audio-visual.

The other big misunderstanding about dyslexics is that they don't hear the sounds of the letters, that they don't have phonemic awareness. That is not true. And for much the same reason that it isn't what a dyslexic sees that is the source of the problem.

The human mind tries to make sense out of what comes in through its senses. It automatically ignores the position of the head and tail of a dog for identification purposes. It judges size of objects not by the amount of space it takes up on the back of the retina but by the relationship it has to other objects within the field of vision. The television and movie special effects people use this phenomenon to create new "realities" as in the movie, *Honey, I Shrunk the Kids*. This is the reason I give for three out of four reading experts in a car misreading a street sign that said KOVAL as ROYAL. It was night. It was in Las Vegas. We had just minutes before driven by Caesar's Palace. Wham. Here is a street sign. There is no word KOVAL in the English Language. The name, yes. Word, no. And because KOVAL was not a name frequently encountered by at least three of us, our minds simple construed the K as R and the V as Y.

Not only does the human mind, especially the dyslexic mind, misconstrue letters and letter order, it does the same with sounds. This I have demonstrated time and time again to teachers that the ability to hear specific phonemic sounds is not important. It's the combination of phonemes, the patterns of phonemes within the context of the intonation, the tone, volume, and phrases surrounding the phonemes that produce the translation of soundwaves into words within the human mind. Sorry about the academic language. I apologize. To help you understand what I'm talking about, I'll give you something you can duplicate if you have a tape recorder. Carefully record the non-word: *sbrattle*. It might not be too easy for you to say. But if there were a word *brattle* and we said it was Pop*'s brattle*, all you have to do is take out the pop and you have *sbrattle* left. Record the word as I have done.

What I love to do is prove to teachers that their ability to hear phonemes is predicated on their experience with words and letters, not with the sounds themselves. Even our legendary Professor Higgins would most likely fail this test. What I do is to tell my audience that I want them to spell a simple little non-word to test their ability to hear sounds. I ask them not to say, "What did you say?" or "Did you say _____? I ask them to focus their attention on the word that I will play from the recorder at the count of three. I say, "One, two, three." SBRATTLE! The spellings: Well, the most common is SPRATTLE. The second most common is BRATTLE! Others are SPRADDLE, STRADDLE, and BRADDLE. After I tell them what the word was and show them the correct spelling, then and only then can they hear the S-B-R consonant blend in the word SBRATTLE. What happens is that each person's computer brain slightly adjusts what it actually hears (the jargon is processes) to fit the situation.

This is why if somebody from Boston asks me, "WAY'r kin AH pah'k muh KAH?", I understand him as saying, "Where can I park my car?" That is why you can take the words: Wants pawn tom dare worst tree bars, and if you pronounced them with the proper intonation everybody will understand what you said as being: Once upon a time there were three bears. Try it!

Part IV, Chapter 26

Computers can be part of the solution, but beware of GIGO: Garbage In; Garbage Out.

WE ARE RAPIDLY ENTERING an age in which computers will be part of almost everybody's daily life. And computers are great. This book couldn't have been written without one. At least, not the way it is. Schools and homes will soon be connected with the internet. We will all soon have access to all kinds of information from all over the world. But that access will be meaningful only to those who can read.

Our schools are buying more and more computers. More and more they will be relying on Computer Managed Instruction (MAI). Perhaps, that is the way it should be. Computers can free up teachers for individualized instruction. Computers can also provide individualized instruction, but again, unless the programs provide good synthesized speech, the ability to read is a pre-requisite. So is the ability to spell.

What about spell check? Won't that solve our students' spelling problems? Hardly. You have to be a very good speller for it to be of any real help. Try running the word sighkiatryst through spell check. All it says is that it isn't in the dictionary. You just have to know that "sighkiatryst" starts with the letter *p* followed by *sych*. It will then correct *psychkiatryst* to *psychiatrist*. But I use spell check. I use it a lot. Why? Well, one obvious reason is that I make typos. The first time through this paragraph I had three l's in the word spelling. Spell check catches that. But spell check doesn't catch my typing *you* for *your* or *shift* for *shirt*. The spell checking abilities of computers is handy, but it is not a real help to dyslexics who haven't been taught. If anything, it's a horrible frustration.

Today, the big move is to computers in the classroom. Everybody is scrambling for more and more hardware. Everybody is searching for decent software. It seems to me that the craze for computers will ebb and our special education classrooms will be left with computers that are used mainly for their games and as rewards for work well done.

I hope I'm wrong. There are many good things that computers can do. But I wonder sometimes if teachers themselves can't do all the good things that computers do.

Computers have PATIENCE. I think teachers can acquire this virtue if they don't already possess it.

Computers don't pass judgment. They simply give automatic feedback, right or wrong. Sometimes built-in remarks such as "GOOD TRY!" or "SORRY, TRY AGAIN" appear on a computer's screen. Teachers are known to say things like that too, but let's go back to the automatic feedback concept. Do teachers use this? Sometimes. But not enough. Where it is used most frequently is when the teacher uses flash cards. Here, even though the teacher may only be asking one student to respond -- all (or almost all) of the students will respond mentally with an answer. The student who is called upon has his/her answer verified. The rest of the students then automatically compare their answer with the correct answer given.

Most of us remember making our own flash cards whether for math tables or for learning vocabulary in our French, Spanish, Latin or German classes. Some of us even made fact flash cards in preparation for studying for finals in history, science, law, etc. in college. It is the immediate feedback that works. This is the educationally operative feature of computers.

Now, what we as teachers can do is: (1) have a computer terminal for each student, (2) buy the best software available, (3) create our own software. Since most critics of educational software agree that good software for the teaching of reading and spelling to students with special needs is almost non-existent (Oh, do I hope I'm wrong or they're wrong!), what is left is creating your own computer software.

Or, if you don't have computers, you can still create your own software and be the computer that your students are plugged into. I first started thinking about this when I first created AVKO's *Sequential Spelling*.

By now, most of your readers should be familiar with the technique. But in case you may have forgotten, it goes like this:

1. You give the word, use it in a sentence, and give the word one last time.

2. The students write the word.

3. Then just like a computer, you give the correct spelling. Preferably by calling out the letters as you write them on the chalkboard or show them using the overhead projector.

4. Now, if any students made a mistake, they correct the mistake right then and there.

When I was teaching and developing Sequential Spelling in the Flint Public Schools, some of my students complained: "Do we have to do this every day?" So, I did something that I rarely do. I gave them a choice. You should never (well, almost never) give students a choice, but I did. I told them they could have the ten minute *AVKO Sequential Spelling* drill every day or a traditional list of twenty-five words to learn and be graded by 100% being an A; miss one, a B; miss two, a C; miss four or more an E. For some strange reason, my students chose Sequential Spelling. They preferred my giving an A if they correct all their mistakes. Forget to correct one mistake and it's an E.

They even liked my way of mastery testing. For example, when I tested their ability to spell the -at, -ats, -atted, -atting, -atty, -atties, -atter, -atters, -attered, -attering, -attery, -atteries, -attle, -attles, -attled, -attling, -attler, and -attlers rimes, they didn't have to worry about correctly spelling the onsets. That is, the beginning letters.

See samples on following page.

My Test Sheet	Student Answer Sheet
1. flat	1. fl_____
2. splatter	2. spl_____
3. platters	3. pl_____
4. flattery	4. fl_____
5. cattle	5. c_____

When I tested on their ability to spell the onsets, they didn't have to worry about the rimes.

My Test Sheet	Student Answer Sheet
1. flat	1. ____at
2. splatter	2. ____atter
3. platters	3. ____atters
4. flattery	4. ____attery
5. cattle	5. ____attle

However, *AVKO Sequential Spelling* doesn't really cover the scrunched up words and tricky words very well. My students were constantly misspelling words such as *there, their, and they're*. One student of mine had completely given up on trying to tell which was which and spelled all of them "thair."

At that time, I had developed an AVKO Teacher's Manual and started using what I called at the time, *Spoken Dialect Translation Exercises*. And that's really what they were. But titles like that really frighten many teachers. Now, I just call the process *Sentence Dictation for Spelling Improvement*. What I did was to dictate the whole sentence, sometimes repeating it four or five times. After all the students had written the sentence I had dictated, I then wrote the sentence on the board. It worked except that it seemed to take too much time out of the class period. And, for some of my students, it was just too hard. For example, one of my students had tested out at 1.8 reading level and he was in the 10th grade! Although he could handle Sequential Spelling and was really progressing fast, he wasn't ready for all the "big" words all at one time. So, what I did for him was to use the principle of the sentences but have them pre-printed with big spaces for the words I wanted spelled. (See Fig. 1) When I read the sentences, everybody read along with me. It was helpful to the slow students. They weren't just left alone in the corner to struggle doing an exercise containing words they couldn't read. They were participating with the entire class. I was the computer. A very sophisticated computer, one that could speak *with intonation*, with rhythm, and with expression. My students would fill in the blanks and then I would give them the correct spelling. I also used the technique to build in reviews. Once an "outlaw" word (such as *wasn't* or *knew*) was introduced in an exercise, I would always use a blank for it even though the lesson might be on the troublesome "TOOZ" (*to, too, two*) or *then/than* or whatever.

What I ended up doing, because I'm basically lazy is assigning my students to write as homework four sentences every single day using words I assign. The best sentences I put into my dictation exercises -- **and give them credit**.

The following is just one day's dictation. My series for teaching the "THAYRZ" runs for three weeks, i.e., 15 consecutive lessons. By the time they are finished, my L.D. students know the difference and do much better than the regular students in our school on spelling these words correctly.

Fig. 1
The "THAYRZ" -- Lesson Four
1. Do you ("NOH") _____ Jack and Betty? Have you ever been to ("THAYR") _____ house?
2. ("NOH") _____, I don't ("NOH") _____ them. I heard that ("THAYR") _____ good ("FRENZ") _____ of yours.
3. How many of your friends and ("THAYR") _____ friends are going to be ("THAYR") _____?
4. I think ("THAYR") _____ will be about five of each at ("THAYR") _____ party.

Normal commercial exercises on the "THAYRZ" would consist of maybe ten sentences to be completed by the students by themselves at their seats. After the exercises are completed, the teacher would correct them and hand them back in a day or two with grades on them. The students just take a look at the grade and throw the papers away. Learning rarely takes place this way. With computers, the students do learn. An exercise on the "THAYRZ" on a computer gives the students instant feedback. And they generally learn. So, why not use the same techniques that work with computers? You can be your own computer for your class. You can let the students plug into you and receive the correct answers immediately and learn.

If you like my concept but just don't have the time to be creative, you might be interested in trying one of the following: *The Tricky Words Levels A, B, and C, Apostrophes Made Easy, The "IT-ss" and the "TOOZ" Made Easy*. Also, much the same concept is expressed in my Reading Improvement through SITDOWN, AVKO Great Idea Reprint #634 which costs less than a dollar. Readers mentioning this book, can receive it free if they send a stamped self-addressed envelope.

In re-reading what I have written, I discovered that I forgot two rather important things. One, is how my wife Ann should be in the *Guiness Book of World's Records*. There are many women who have captured live animals. Not quite so many who have captured one with one hand, their left hand. When we narrow the capturing down to those who have captured one-handed an animal inside a house while sitting down reading a book in the bathroom, I think that eliminates all but Ann. While quietly reading, she had noticed in the corner of her eye something brown move. She reached down with her left hand and, like a magician, came up with a rabbit, a rabbit that our cat had dragged in. "Don," she called, "Come in here, I've got something to show you." I went into the bathroom and she smiled and handed me the rabbit. All I had to do was to carry it out of the house and past our German Shepard's nose and release it.

The other thing I forgot to tell was the reason why I wear a Basque beret. It isn't because I'm an artist, although I suppose I could lay claim to being one. It's so easy to do today. And it's not because I am trying to hide the fact that I'm bald. Although the beret does keep my head warm. I started wearing the beret as the result of coming out of a session at the Michigan Reading Association's annual conference and seeing in the shop window a sign that said: BASQUE BERET, 12.95. It suddenly dawned on me that not one of my students would be able to read those two words. In fact, probably over half Flint's high school graduates wouldn't be able to read those two words, let alone spell them. So, I went in and paid the outrageous price for the Basque beret. I put it on as a symbol of those words that follow phonic patterns that are never taught in our schools, but should be.

Nearly everywhere I speak I put on the chalkboard or overhead the words ASQUE ERET before I begin my lecture, inservice, or whatever. When I'm finished and ask for questions, there generally are none. Then, I point to the ASQUE ERET and state that no one ever bothered to ask about those words. Why? Isn't the answer obvious? How do you ask about ASQUE ERET without the possibility of being laughed at or exposing your ignorance? Then I compare their hesitancy about asking to the hesitancy of students to ask questions involving words. Once I add capital B's to both ASQUE and ERET and show BASQUE BERET, the audience of teachers usually understand my point. There are certain phonic patterns that exist in our language that need to be taught. The -sque (-sk) pattern occurs in words such as masque, masquerade, grotesque, brusque, bisque, and picturesque. The -et having the "AY" sound occurs in hundreds of words from beret and buffet to Chevrolet. So I end my lecture with the statement that I will continue to wear my Basque beret until I can find one urban public high school in which half the students can both read and spell those two words. If and when I find one, I will take my Basque beret, run it through a blender with a few jalepeno peppers, and drink it.

I hope someday that a school system will teach all its students to read and spell so well that not only will I be forced to eat my words but to drink my beret as well.

<u>Appendix</u>

This contains many miscellaneous items, some of which may not be of any interest to you. To help you decide which you may wish to skip and which you want to read, we have a special table of contents.

Appendix item #1.

☺ Organizations whose goals include the offering of information concerning dyslexia.

The Three Organizations that AVKO Believes Are Your Best Bet for Help.

AVKO Educational Research Foundation
3084 W. Willard Road, Clio, MI 48420
(810) 686-9283   FAX (810) 686-1101

The Family Literacy Center, Indiana University, 2805 E. 10th St, Smith Research Center, Suite 150 Bloomington, IN 47408
(800) 759-4723   FAX (812) 855-4220

Orton Dyslexia Society
Chester Building, Suite 382, Baltimore, MD 21286-2044
(410) 296-0232   (800) ABCD123

Other Excellent Organizations Which May Be of Help to You

Adult Learning Disabilities Association
510 West Hastings Street, Suite 1322 Vancouver, British Columbia, Canada V6B 1L8 (604) 683-5554   FAX (604) 683-2380

American Council of Rural Special Education (ACRES)
221 Milton Bennion Hall, University of Utah
Salt Lake City, UT 84112

Continued on the next three pages

Association on Higher Education & Disability (AHEAD)
PO Box 21192 Columbus, OH 43221
(614) 488-4972

The Attention Deficit Information Network, Inc. (AD-IN)
475 Hillside Avenue, Needham, MA 02194
(617) 455-0585

Children and Adults with Attention Deficit Disorders (CHADD)
499 NW 70th Ave, Suite 308, Plantation, FL 33317
(305) 587-3700   FAX: (305) 587 -4599

Dyslexia Research Institute, Inc.
4745 Centerville Road, Tallahassee, FL 32308
(904) 893-2216   FAX (904) 893-2440

Irlen Institute for Perceptual & Learning Development
5380 Village Road, Long Beach, CA 90808
(310) 496-2550 (Best source of information concerning Scotopic
Sensitivity Syndrome which affects some dyslexics, myself included.)

Learning Disabilities Association of America (LDA)
4156 Library Road, Pittsburgh, PA 15234
(412) 341-1515   (412) 341-8077

Learning Disabilities Association of Canada
323 Chapel Street, Suite 200, Ottawa, Ontario, Canada K1N 7Z2
(613) 238-5721   FAX: (613) 235-5391

The Learning Disabilities Network
72 Sharp Street, Suite A-2, Hingham, MA 02043
(617) 340-5605

National Adult Literacy and Learning Disabilities Center
1875 Connecticut Ave, NW, Suite 800, Washington, DC 20009-1202
(202) 884-8185   FAX (202) 884-8422

National Association for Adults with Special Learning Needs
PO Box 716, Bryn Mawr, PA 19010
(610) 535-8336   FAX (610) 525-8337

National Catholic Office for Persons with Disabilities
PO Box 29113, Washington DC 20017
(202) 529-2933   (202) 529-4678

National Center for Learning Disabilities
381 Park Avenue South, New York, NY 10016
(212) 545-7510

National Learning Disabilities Network
82 South Townline Road, Sandusky, MI 48471-9723
(810) 648-2125   FAX (810) 648-4418

The Rebus Institute
1499 Bayshore Blvd, Suite 146, Burlingame, CA 94010
(415) 697-7424   FAX (415) 607-3734

Clearinghouse on Adult Education and Literacy
400 Maryland Ave., SW, Washington, DC 20202-7240
(202) 205-9996   FAX (202) 205-8973

Clearinghouse on Disability Information US Dept Educ
Room 3132 Switzer Bldg, Washington, DC 20202-2524
(202) 205-8723   (202) 205-8241

ERIC Clearinghouse on Reading, English, & Cmm. Indiana Univ
Smith Research Center, Suite 150, Bloomington, IN 47408-2798
(812)855-5847   (800) 759-4723

Institute for the Study of Adult Literacy, Penn. State Univ.
204 Calder Way, Suite 209, University Park, PA 16801-4756
(814) 863-3777   FAX (814) 863-6108

Appendix item #2.   Improvement English

Report submitted to Flint Board of Education.

The following report was submitted by me on behalf of the Professional Study Committee which had been established by the first Master Teacher Contract between the Flint Education Association (FEA) and the Flint Public Schools.

To: The Flint Board of Education and the Flint Education Association.

From: The FEA members of the Professional Study Committee (PSC) as established by the Master Teacher Contract.

Section C of Article XVII states: The PSC is empowered to appoint subcommittees composed of teachers and administrators to study and report upon *any* mutually agreed upon subjects.

Section E of Article XVII states: Subject of study by subcommittees shall include but not be limited to:

1. Discipline policy.
2. Evaluation of Teachers.
3. Development of Curriculum.

While we recognize the right of the administrative members of the PSC to *not agree* to the establishment of any particular proposed subcommittee, we believe it is a clear cut violation of the Master Teacher Contract to rigidly oppose the formation of any subcommittee that would study and report on:

1. any area already covered in part by the Master Teacher Contract
2. any area that would or could be a negotiable area.
3. any area that would be a specific area in the development of curriculum.
4. any area that does not affect all or nearly all teachers.

Because we have not been able to resolve these matters and because we believe that they should be resolved one way or the other before the next school year ends, we are asking you to resolve them.

Since it would be presumptuous on our part to state the reasons why the administrative component of our committee have taken the above mentioned position, we feel that you should ask them to explain to you why they have unanimously opposed the formation of every subcommittee that we have proposed. If you believe their reasons to be valid we would like the opportunity to refute them.

SPECIAL NOTE TO MEMBERS OF THE BOARD OF EDUCATION.

While the Master Teacher Contract does not restrict your choice as to the members you appoint, we would like to take this opportunity to suggest that the three members you appoint should all be principals. This should not be construed as a criticism of Mr. Frosty. He has been most cooperative and a very valuable member of the PSC. However, since the reports of the PSC subcommittees are filed by its administrative co-chairmen to the Assistant Superintendent, it does seem strange to have the Assistant Superintendent filing a report to himself.

After Note: There no longer is a Professional Study Committee in the Flint Public Schools. The letter was never answered. Even the teachers' union did not respond to the letter.

Appendix item #3. Improvement English

The following is a copy of a proposal I made to the administration of the Flint Public Schools. It includes the results of the testing of all the students at Northwestern High School. No action on this proposal was taken unless you consider the adoption of a myriad of English courses from "Man and the Motor Car" to "Girl Talk" as being somehow related to this. Not one of the following suggested courses was ever implemented.

IMPROVEMENT ENGLISH

I. To be a required subject for all first semester sophomores for the following reasons:

  A. **90.8%** of the Flint Northwestern high school sophomores are **below 50** percentile in one or more of the following areas: reading comprehension, vocabulary, capitalization, grammar, spelling.

  B. Only 4.6% had scores of at least 65 percentile or higher in all the above areas.

  C. No student had scores of 85 percentile or higher in all the above areas.

I. Objectives of the course:

  A. To bring reading levels up to a minimum of the 9th grade level.

    1. 47% of the College Prep students at the end of their 10th year were reading below the 9th grade level. Only 19% of the College Prep students who had participated in the programmed learning experiment conducted by Mr. McCabe were reading below the 9th grade level at the end of their 10th year.

    2. 86% of the Non-College students at the end of their 10th year were reading below the 9th grade level. Only 50% of the Non-College students who had participated in the programmed learning

experiment conducted by Mr. McCabe were reading below the 9th grade level at the end of their 10th year.

3. 64% of the students at the end of their 10th year were reading below the 9th grade level as compared to 30% of the students who had participated in the programmed learning experiment.

B. To bring spelling levels up to the 9th grade level.

1. 30% of the College Prep students were below the 9th grade level in spelling at the end of their 10th year as compared to only 16% of those who had participated in the programmed learning experiment.

2. 80% of the Non-College Prep students were spelling below the 9th grade level as compared to 58% of those who had participated in the programmed learning experiment.

3. 55% of the Non-College Prep students at the end of their 10th year were BELOW THE 7TH GRADE LEVEL in spelling as compared to only 29% of those who had participated in the programmed learning experiment.

Suggested Approaches to Solving the Problem.

I. Minimum standards of achievement tests in 6th grade, 8th and 9th.

A. Students failing minimum achievement standards in any area will be required to take an improvement course designed to help him/her attain adequate proficiency in that area.

B. Specialized courses using multi-level programmed materials will be used.

II. Individualized Curriculum in the Language Arts Area.

    A. 1/2 semester courses with final grades given at present marking period times.

    B. Specialized courses to meet individual needs.

        1. Introduction to high school study (Required of all incoming sophomores.)

            a. Dictionary skills. Each student to be issued a dictionary to be turned in at the end of his school career.

            b. How to study (SRA)

            c. How to listen (SRA)

            d. How to take notes (SRA)

            e. How to increase reading speed and comprehension (SRA)

        2. Reading Improvement. May be taken along with another English course by any student. Should be required of all who do not reach 9th grade level at the end of 1st 15 weeks.

        3. Elements of Traditional Grammar using a programmed text (not Warriner's) and required of all those scoring below 65 percentile. Need not be repeated by those who fail.

        4. Elements of Modern Grammar to be required of all those who fail #3 but may be taken as an elective.

        5. Problems in Politically[1] and Socially Correct Usage with emphasis on equipping students with

---

[1]The term *politically correct* wasn't in usage then. I used just the phrase socially correct in the original document. I only added the phrase *politically correct* to better demonstrate the concept presented.

the options of choosing the more appropriate choice of written or oral patterns. If one knows only one type of speech, one has no choice.

6. Spelling Improvement I through VII to be required by all students who fail to reach 9th grade level. Must be "repeated" until satisfactory level (as determined by teacher, student, parent, and counselor) is achieved. Grade of C is virtually automatic regardless of achievement.

7. Perfect Spelling for Good Spellers. This is also tied into Vocabulary Development.

8. Basic Composition I & II. Only I is required; II is optional. Using SRA programmed materials.

9. Advanced Composition. (SRA-High School Kit.)

10. Creative writing. Elective.

11. Journalism. Elective.

12. Debate. Elective will fulfill speech requirement.

13. Public Speaking. Elective. Will fulfill speech requirement.

14. Speech Improvement. Required except of those who take #12 or #13.

15. Vocabulary Development I & II. Required of all. Use of individualized, programmed multi-level materials designed to improve word attack skills and make students more word conscious.

16. Speed Reading. Optional. Using mechanical aids such as the reading accelerator.

Appendix Item #4: Descriptions of materials I developed especially for dyslexics and their 1995 prices.

Description of the Contents of

The Patterns of English Spelling
8½ x 11, Over 900 pages, $89.95
This is a tool that should be in every library!

Part #	Pattern	Examples			Pages
1	Short Vowels **CVC**	dad cab fit	get dig man	tin rip call	101-162
2	Short Vowels **CVCC**	hand lift salt	went lamp milk	itch path tack	201-282
3	Long Vowels **CV & CVCe**	go fly me	nice note gate	tube Jane time	301-380
4	Long Vowels **CVVC**	raid vein weight	seem read field	roam crawl taught	401-442
5	**W- & -R** Controls	tar/war car/wart sand/wand	for/word forth/worth form/worm	wad/ward wan/warn wasp/warp	501-548
6	Basic Suffixes	er batter en fatten or labor	le battle el tunnel our labour	ful dreadful ible possible able probable	601-691
7	The Ending Y's	destiny privacy geography	simplify therapy monarchy	tricky memory thrifty	701-764

8	Power Suffixes	precious	partially	permission	801-880
		ferocious	initially	compassionate	
		luscious	especially	ignition	
9	Advanced Patterns	technique	chauvinist	fiancée	901-962
		ricochet	bureau	debut	
		surgeon	impartial	compulsion	
10	Prefixes	photograph	synthetic	sympathy	1001-1074
	Suffixes	psychology	euphemism	magnitude	
	Roots	beneficial	unconscious	linguistics	

Alphabetic Index has 92 pages with over 25,000 entries. See sample entries below.

Word	page	LD	
			LD stands for **L**evel of **D**ifficulty on a scale of 1.00 to 21.00
call	<u>147</u>	1.55	See next page for the -all family (rime!)
called	147	2.40	
caller	634		
calling	147	2.45	
callisthenics	807		
callous*	888		* means there is a homophone.
calls	147	5.25	
callus*	160		* means there is a homophone.
calm	119	9.35	

Sample Page from The Patterns of English Spelling

Reduced from 8½ x 11 to fit this page

ALL TALL (TAW'L) Family

See Rhyming Families Awl Crawl & Aul Paul on p. 416
-alled also rhymes with -ald BALD Family p. 240

AW'l all	AW'l-z	AW'l-d	AW ling	AW lee	AW lur
hall	halls				
call	calls	called	calling		caller
tall					taller
fall	falls		falling		
wall	walls	walled	walling	Wally	
ball	balls	balled	balling		
small					

Power Vocabulary

stall	stalls	stalled	stalling		
install	installs	installed	installing	installment	installation
forestall	forestalls	forestalled	forestalling		
recall	recalls	recalled	recalling		
overcall	overcalls	overcalled	overcalling		
gall	galls	galled	galling		
enthrall	enthralls	enthralled	enthralling		

More ALL words

rainfall	waterfall	pitfall	nightfall	snowfall	overall
pratfall	eyeball	cannonball	softball	oddball	meatball
football	baseball	basketball	snowball	mall	paddleball
pinball	racquetball	screwball	downfall	tetherball	volleyball
gumball	hairball	hardball	highball	kickball	know-it-all

Difficulty Levels on scale of 1.00 to 21.00: all 1.30, small 2.85
Dolch Words: all shall
Exception: shall. (The word *shall* is pronounced: "shal," or "shel")
Spelling Demon: football
Homophones: balled/bald, hall/haul
Other Related Families: -ller, p. 634; -lly, p. 703; -llow, p. 684

Sequential Spelling I through VII (8.95 each)
Each book contains 180 lessons, 1 for each day in the school year,
enough for seven years.

● Utilizes immediate student self-correction.
● Builds from easier words of a word family to important power
words that build self-confidence. Each of the seven levels contains
180 spelling lessons that teach phonics through the backdoor of
spelling. Students learn the patterns without having to memorize
rules.
● Sequences two ways: (1) Vertically during a single lesson.
(2) Horizontally Monday through Friday.

Sample from Level 1

Monday	Tuesday	Wednesday
all	ball	balls
tall	fall	falls
stall	stalls	stalled
install	installs	installed

Sample from Level 2

end	ends	ended
tend	tends	tended
intend	intends	intended
attend	attends	attended

Sample from Level 3

rain	rains	rained
train	trains	trained
strain	strains	strained
restrain	restrains	restrained

Sample from Level 4

serve	serving	service
reserve	reserving	reservation
preserve	preserving	preservation
conserve	conserving	conservation

Sample from Level 5

include	inclusive	inclusion
exclude	exclusive	exclusion
conclude	conclusive	conclusion
intrude	intrusive	intrusion

Sample from Level 6

democrat	democratic	democracy
aristocrat	aristocratic	aristocracy
diplomat	diplomatic	diplomacy
bureaucrat	bureaucratic	bureaucracy

Sample from Level 7

decorate	decoration	decorative
interrogate	interrogation	interrogative
demonstrate	demonstration	demonstrative
legislate	legislation	legislative

One book is all that is necessary for an entire class!

So what can a parent of a dyslexic do?

1. Send for the Free booklet: *How to Set Up a Community Education Course for Adults whose Children (or Spouses) Have Reading/Spelling Problems.*

2. Read and present it to a school board member. Show the school board member the offer for the FREE lesson plans for the course.

3. Purchase for yourself the companion books: *If it is to be it is up to me to do it* (Student book, 9.95) and *If it is to be it is up to me to help* (Parent's book, 9.95).

Order from:

AVKO Educational Research Foundation
3084 W. Willard Road
Clio, MI 48420-7801

Telephone: (810) 686-9283   or FAX: (810) 686-1101